Empowerment and Participation: Power, influence and control in contemporary health care

Also published by Quay Books:

Empowerment and the Health Service User, volume two
edited by James Dooher and Richard Byrt

Dedicated to the memory of Davies

Empowerment and Participation: Power, influence and control in contemporary health care

volume one

James Dooher and Richard Byrt

Quay
Books

Mark Allen
Publishing Ltd

Quay Books Division, Mark Allen Publishing Limited, Jesses Farm,
Snow Hill, Dinton, Wiltshire, SP3 5HN

British Library Cataloguing-in-Publication Data
A catalogue record is available for this book

© Mark Allen Publishing Ltd 2002
ISBN 1 85642 207 0

Printed in the UK by The Cromwell Press, Trowbridge, Wiltshire

Contents

List of contributors

Jayne Breeze BA (Hons) M Med Sci, Cert Ed, RMN works as a Nurse Lecturer at the University of Sheffield.

Larry Butler founded and developed Survivors' Poetry Scotland. He recently completed a feasibility study for the Greater Glasgow Health Board on the idea of 'Arts on Prescription' and is helping to create an arts/eco village.

Richard Byrt RMN, RNMH, PhD is Clinical/Education Facilitator at Arnold Medium Secure Unit, Nottinghamshire Healthcare NHS Trust, and the School of Nursing and Midwifery, De Montfort University.

Gerry Carton BA (Hons), Postgraduate Cert Psycho-Social Interventions, RMN, RNMH, RCNT, Cert Ed, RNT, Cert Research, Dip Research is Head of Education and Training, Nottinghamshire Healthcare NHS Trust.

Mel Chevannes BA (Hons), MA, PhD, RGN, RM, RHV, Teachers Cert RHVT is Dean of the School of Health and Director of Health Service Provision at the University of Wolverhampton.

John R Cutcliffe RMN, RGN, BSc (Hons), PhD is Assistant Professor of Nursing at the University of Alberta, Canada.

James Dooher RMN, MA, FHE, Cert Ed, Dip HCR is Senior Lecturer and Pathway Leader for Mental Health at De Montfort University and Clinical Coach for Leicestershire and Rutland Healthcare Trust.

Sue Evans MSc is Head of Final Performance at North Bristol NHS Trust.

Jackie Green Principal Lecturer in Health Promotion at Leeds Metropolitan University and Head of the Centre for Health Promotion Research and also Editor-in-Chief of *Promotion and Education*.

Mark RD Johnson is Professor of Diversity in Health and Social Care at Mary Seacole Research Centre, De Montfort University, Leicester.

Deenesh Khoosal MB, BCh, LLM (RCS), LLM (RCP), BAO (Royal College of Surgeons and Physicians, Ireland), MRCPsyche, FRC Psyche is a Consultant Psychiatrist at the Leicester General Hospital and Clinical Teacher for the Leicester University Medical School.

Judith Reece MA, BA (Hons), BA (Nursing education), RMN, RGN is a Lecturer in Mental Health Nursing at the Open University, UK.

Ray Rowden SRN, RMN, Onc NC, MHSM, Hon D Univ (Kingston) is Visiting Professor of Nursing and Clinical Management at the University of York and a Specialist Adviser for the Health Select Committee, House of Commons.

Sally Rudge RMN, RNMH, BA (Hons), MSc, PG Dip Psychol, Dip Psychol (Open), ACBS is a Community Mental Health Nurse and BPS registered psychologist.

Mike Saks is Pro-Vice Chancellor at the University of Lincoln and is a member of the Regional Management Board of the Trent Focus for Research and Development in Primary Care and the Leicester Health Action Zone Board.

Keith Tones is Emeritus Professor of Health Promotion at Leeds Metropolitan University.

Carrie White is Branch Manager of WISH (Women in Secure Hospitals) and works as a sessional psychotherapist in a therapeutic community.

Lawrence Whyte MA, BA (Hons), RMN, RGN, Cert Ed is a Mental Health/Nurse Educator, who has worked mainly in developing and teaching courses for nurses in secure settings.

Acknowledgements

The authors and editors would like to offer their sincere appreciation to the people, groups, colleagues and organisations without whom, this volume would never exist. A real team effort, thank you. You know who you are. In particular:

Mike Akester
The Byrt family
Leslie Corlett
Millicent Dooher
Elizabeth Dooher
Allyson Evans
Les Gallop
Jeanette Johnson
Jeanette Johnson
Richard Jones
Chris Lomas
Tracey Preston
Jules Mann
Helen Millar
Julie Repper
Ali Sansom
Flick Schofield
David Ward
Adrian Webb
Gerald Wistow

The editors would like to acknowledge, with thanks, the following for granting copyright permission to publish material from work previously published elsewhere:

* Blackwell Science Publications for copyright permission to publish material in *Chapter 6*, previously published in Breeze J, Repper J (1998) Struggling for control: the care experiences of 'difficult' patients in mental health services. *J Adv Nurs* **28**(6): 1300–11; and Breeze J (1998) Can paternalism be justified in mental health care? *J Adv Nurs* **28**(2): 260–5.

❖ IBC UK Conferences Limited for copyright permission to publish material in *Chatper 15*, previously published in: Evans S (2000) Managing Complaints. In: IBC UK Conferences Limited (2000) *Involving Users in Clinical Governance Working with Users to Provide a Quality Service. LH183. Conference Handbook for One Day Conference*. 31 March 2000 at The Marlborough Hotel, London.

Our thanks to Tamzin Ewers and Binkie Mais at Quay Books, the external reviewer of this book and all the contributors for their varied and interesting chapters, which have increased our understanding of empowerment and participation.

We would also like to thank Kath Sanders, Maeve Holms, the library staff at De Montfort University and Leicester University, Jenny Dunhill, Blackwell Science Publishing, Laura Beachus, IBC UK Conferences, Leicestershire Partnership NHS Trust and Nottinghamshire Healthcare NHS Trust.

All royalties from this publication will be donated to Rethink (previously The National Schizophrenia Fellowship) and Marie Curie Cancer Care.

James Dooher, Richard Byrt
September 2002

Foreword

Using empowerment as a healthcare strategy to promote health

Many years ago, the famous sociologist Parsons (1951) described the 'sick role' as a condition where the person in a state of ill health undergoes a loss of power. In order to obtain help, and undergo healing, the patient or 'user' must both want to get better, and also be prepared to 'follow instructions' from the health professional charged with their care. In return for this, the sick person is allowed to derogate from some of their other social responsibilities and expectations (such as staying off work). Some commentators have discussed whether it is the adoption of the sick role that causes the loss of power, or whether the loss of power might be a symptom or cause of ill-health. Clearly, the fastest way to regain control and self-efficacy is to recover the healthy state — but here lies a chicken-and-egg conundrum. The chapters in this book and its companion volume explore the issues around these contested role states, and through greater understanding may reduce the possibility of the 'healer' causing unintended harm, encouraging holistic healing. In a society structured on inequality, of which sickness is merely one of the more easily measured manifestations, this book also raises interesting questions about accountability and ethical practice.

It is important in any transaction, or joint activity, such as healing or caring, to pay attention to the role of all the 'actors' in the situation. This includes both the patient and the clinical professional, and any carers. It may well be that despite personal feelings of inadequacy or hierarchy, the individual possesses more competence or power than they realise. Indeed, even the right to derogate from social responsibility, or act 'irresponsibly', may be a form of power that can be used. Equally, paying some attention to and reflecting on one's own characteristics and behaviour may create a more effective or 'better' healer and carer. In order to engage in this process, it is necessary to consider precisely what is meant by 'participation' and 'empowerment'. As the chapters which follow demonstrate, there are many theories and political or ideological positions and groups in this arena of debate. These are debates that many of the social sciences have engaged in — but they are not irrelevant to healthcare practice. Hopefully, the reader will find that the opening chapters provide a broad and clear review of the principal models, and their implications for the practitioner.

A particular area of concern is the danger of cultural specificity. This, of course, may be challenged in practice through the medium of user (or 'client') involvement, but even that concept might be challenged as Eurocentric, compared to a more holistic model of social and societal involvement in caring. As the contributions demonstrate, it is necessary to have some knowledge of the history of participation to engage with these debates. However, the National Service Frameworks (NSFs) and other new NHS structures such as the PALS (Patient Advocacy Liaison Services) now assume that such reflection and development is ongoing across the health services. It is therefore incumbent on all healthcare practitioners to be able to discuss the issue intelligently, and to have some alternative models to fall back on in their own practice.

Most of the models and examples presented draw on the mental health sector where, indeed, probably most of the discussion and development of models of empowerment and active patient-hood have taken place since at least the days of Foucault. Nevertheless, issues of social conditioning, stigma, exclusion, and the debate over the balance between care and control have a wider applicability in other more obviously 'organic' areas of disease and disability. We may, for example, examine the question of maternity and pregnancy (not a disease, but a condition which often requires clinical and caring input) and the role of the feminist or natural childbirth movements, leading more recently to Government policy in *Changing Childbirth*. Recent Government publications have given explicit recognition to the role of the 'expert patient', and note that today's patients with chronic diseases need not be mere recipients of care but can also become key decision makers and, indeed, inform service planning at a wider level (DoH, 2001). The task force recognised that those who use services have very variable experiences, and only by bringing a mixture of users on board can improvements be made to attain the level of the best experiences.

Nevertheless, we should not fall into the trap of assuming that all users or consumers (or even those who do not at present access the services) want the same thing. Alternative therapies are attractive to some, as Saks suggests (*Chapter 3*), although in the UK and Europe as in Asia, the rise of allopathic or so-called 'western' medical models has been inexorable. In the interests of all, the critical issue is one of regulation and quality control — which to be most effective, in alternative or conventional therapy, requires the active involvement, empowerment, and use of the users themselves.

The chapters which follow provide a way into these debates, informing and stimulating future generations of healthcare professionals (and also those who are now established in their careers) to reflect on their practice, and consider the many ways in which their clients may be excluded. This volume lays out a number of the key dimensions and mechanisms of exclusion, including medicalisation (the rise of the hegemony of biomedicine, described by Saks, *Chapter 3*) and the imposition of mental health legislation (Whyte and Carton, *Chapter 12*), through age (Rudge, *Chapter 9*; Khoosal, *Chapter 10*) as well as by educational level, social status, health and disease. Indeed, even access to decision-making about research can be a significant issue (Cutcliffe, *Chapter 13*), as those of us who espouse the 'social action' model in research to involve users themselves in creating knowledge and 'expertise'. It is also important to consider what may be learned not only from 'good practice' but by examining 'bad practices' as suggested by Rowden (*Chapter 11*). Even senior levels of management may fall foul of the system. It is perhaps as well to conclude by considering that we all may find ourselves with the roles reversed — and how we should wish to be participants in decision making for our own health. Do we not owe our users no less?

Mark RD Johnson
Professor of Diversity in Health and Social Care
Mary Seacole Research Centre
De Montfort University, Leicester
April 2002

References

Department of Health (2001) *The Expert Patient: A new approach to chronic disease management for the 21st century*. DoH, London; http://www.doh.gov.uk/healthinequalities

Parsons T (1951) *The Social System*. The Free Press, Glencoe

1

Power

James Dooher and Richard Byrt

When a person becomes ill and seeks professional help, they lose aspects of their independence and hand over some, if not all the responsibilities for the restoration of their health, to another. This move from a state of independence to a state of dependence may involve a complex change of perceived social role and status within society.

Despite the recognition from generations of observers and governments (Beveridge, 1948; Parsons, 1957; Goffman, 1961; Brooker and Repper, 1998; Department of Health [DoH] 1971, 1975, 1989, 1991) that this is disempowering, financially costly and generally unwelcome, professionals seem to perpetuate their indispensability to society, and continue to promote covertly the disparities which set them aside from the rest of humanity.

The concept of power in health may be seen as a microcosm of dilemmas faced in society. Power is said to be a pervasive aspect of all human relationships. Power comes in many forms, political, social and economic and there appears to be a direct relationship between the amount of power an individual, group or organisation has, and their ability to achieve their objectives. How much power an individual or group holds, governs how far they are able to put their wishes into practice at the expense of those of others. Inevitably, conflicts in society arise. For those without power, it is a theoretical concept and perhaps something to strive for; for those with power, it seems to be something to hold on to at all costs. The notion of empowering others is perhaps a rather difficult thing to achieve, at a cognitive and practical level. Power may be seen as the ability of an individual, or the members of a group to achieve or promote the interests they hold, yet professionals within the healthcare arena must share their power to be seen as progressive. This is not a wholly altruistic donation as there are a number of primary and secondary gains to be reaped.

When hospital admission and subsequent diagnosis create powerlessness, the victim (often described as the patient, service user or customer) is left feeling angry and humiliated. Lindow (1990) suggests survivors must engage professionals to redress this imbalance, but warns that this may be an uncomfortable and tense process for all concerned. The government has set its agenda of rights and responsibilities for the patient in *Your guide to the NHS* (DoH, 2001), which sets out national standards and services people can expect from the NHS. This chapter examines some of the factors that influence the divisions of power from a macro and micro perspective, drawing upon health, management and social policy theory.

Power and conflict

A major source of frustration is conflict between two opposing motives. When two motives conflict, the satisfaction of one often leads to the frustration of the other.

When power struggles develop, conflicts between the parties arise. They can involve almost any issue, and may become intractable, with individuals or groups on both sides feeling frustrated and disempowered. The denial of a person's sense of self, their security or the legitimacy of his or her group identity often leads to intractable conflicts. Problems arise when one party forces another party to do something that they do not want to do through social, political, and economic domination or oppression (which may be overt or covert).

Disputants often fail to recognise that they usually have a range of options to solve the discord, each with their own advantages and disadvantages. This lack of awareness of available options can cause the pursuit of ineffective confrontation strategies. For example, people may pursue aggressive or even violent resistance strategies, when non-violent action might be more effective.

Faced with a difficult conflict, disputants sometimes overlook the possibility of using negotiation or persuasion to improve the situation, relying instead on force. While threatening to use force is quite inexpensive, carrying out the threats and actually using force can be costly in terms of the consequences. The cost of using force-based threats increases dramatically when the opponent responds to a threat with defiance rather than submission, and the use of force is most likely to occur when the other side has already used force. In this case, the most common reaction is to respond with equal or even greater force. Resentment and retaliation is especially likely when victims of force believe that the use of or type of force used against them was illegitimate.

Individuals, groups or organisations that use forced-based strategies, for example, violence or other aggressive techniques, assume that their opponents will quickly submit to their demands, thereby providing a quick route to successful accomplishment of their goal. This presumption is misplaced, as although the recipient may appear to acquiesce, they will often try to build up their power so that they can retaliate or reverse the decision when the opportunity arises.

In cases where people are subjected to an overwhelming force that they do not have the power to resist, it may be most appropriate to submit and accept defeat; although often the pretence of submission may, in reality, be manipulative, as they are pursuing a deceptive strategy which allows them to avoid complying with those demands. In 1991, Vivien Lindow reported that when patients, or service users have a legitimate complaint about the service they receive, this is often passed off as a symptom of their illness, and if complaints persist, medication may be increased until they cannot speak clearly, or they learn to make only acceptable statements. When people find themselves in situations in which they have no control, they are said to deteriorate into a state of learned helplessness (Seligman, 1973) leading to apathy, loss of interest, passivity and the symptoms of depression.

Individuals, groups, organisations and at its most basic level the family, can build their power base and their ability to pursue (or resist) force-based strategies by building coalitions with others who have complementary interests. Members of these coalitions promise to help each other advance their joint interests and defend themselves from force-based strategies of their opponents. The dynamics within the family itself represent a microcosm of power relationships, and this is particularly evident in the relationship between parents and children.

The role of parenting is a fundamental example of a relationship in which there is unequal balance of power between children and their responsible adults.

This imbalance of power may be exhibited in a range of inter-actions between parents and their children. Patterns of reward and punishment dispensed in disciplinary confrontations, assertion of power such as physical punishment, criticism and threats are all examples of parental power. Other examples seen are maternal deprivation or love withdrawal as a non-physical expression of dis-approval and the withholding of affection and, at the other end of the spectrum, induction, where the power is used for reasoning and focusing on the impact and consequences of the child's actions on others.

Authority

Authority can be seen as the legitimate power of an individual to direct subordinates within the scope of their position. That position may be political, social, economic, spiritual or cultural. Authority is essentially an abstract and conceptual perception of prestige, derived from the cumulative aspects of responsibility, accountability and the power associated with a particular office or position. The term authority is perhaps most commonly associated with organisations and the world of work, where the vested authority is legitimised by some form of organisational structure. This organisational structure provides the framework for the formal distribution of power and the achievement of the organisational mission. There are said to be three forms of authority: line authority, staff authority, and team authority, each of which provides a justifying rationale for the implementation of power.

Line authority is direct supervisory authority from superior to subordinate. Authority flows in a direct chain of command from the top of the organisation to the bottom. With this type of power comes accountability, the professional and legal obligations associated with the hierarchical position. In nursing, this is best represented by the clinical grading structure

Staff authority is more limited, and restricted to the authority to advise. It is often associated with flattened hierarchies, where authority is based on expertise and usually involves advising line managers. Staff members are advisers and counsellors who aid their colleagues in making decisions but do not have the authority to make final decisions themselves. There is often some confusion in staff authority and the difference between role and responsibility. Those with staff authority rely on their charisma, the power of persuasion and their personal reputation to influence their peers, rather than the power of sanctions against other individuals. These roles are often utilised by clinicians involved in service development, such as practice development nurses and nurse advisors.

Team authority is granted to committees or work teams involved in an organisation's daily operations. Work teams are groups of operating employees, usually of equal rank, empowered to plan and organise their own work. Team authority requires minimum supervision, and relies upon the concepts of personal and professional accountability to control the behaviour of the team as a whole, and the individuals within it. At its most effective, individuals utilise the processes of personal and professional reflection to improve their performance and complete their goals.

Professional power

Professional power is the ability to exert influence upon individuals or groups beyond any vested authority, which is derived from position. Personal power could include:

- job knowledge
- personal influence
- interpersonal skills
- the ability to get results
- empathetic ability
- persuasive ability
- physical strength.

French and Raven (1959) identify six sources of power:

- legitimate
- coercive
- reward
- expert
- referent
- information.

Legitimate power is a result of the position a person holds in the organisation's hierarchy. This position power is broader than the ability to reward and punish, as members need to accept the authority of the position.

Coercive power is the threat of sanctions. It is dependent on fear and includes, but is not limited to the ability to dismiss, assign undesirable work, or restriction of movement.

Reward power results in people doing what is asked because they desire positive benefits or rewards. Rewards can be anything a person values (praise, salary increases, and promotion).

Expert power comes from expertise, skill, or knowledge.

Referent power refers to a person who has desirable resources or personal traits. It results in admiration and the desire to emulate.

Information power is based upon the persuasiveness or content of some form of communication and is independent of the influencing individual.

Medical diagnosis is the power doctors have to define and diagnose disease, and to prescribe treatments for the restoration of health. On the face of it this seems perfectly just and proper, however, despite the advantages in providing a framework for reference of evidence-based knowledge and practice, it may be disempowering for those who are diagnosed. This may take the form of taking on a stigmatised role in society, where one loses individuality and is labelled as the illness itself. For example, the parents of a fifteen-year-old boy diagnosed with schizophrenia may feel relief that they are not alone having a child who behaves in this way, but their son may suffer a lifetime of prejudice because of the label that he has acquired. Professionals use diagnoses as a quick way to categorise their clients, often failing to see the real person because of it. The training of doctors, nurses, social workers, etc. is often cited as one of the main promoters of professional power, and it is only fairly recently that the governing bodies have recognised the need to engage service users in the process of curriculum design and delivery (UKCC, 1999). Pembroke (1991) suggested that people with direct experience are the only experts and should be involved in de-training health workers. If service user's expertise is derived only from their experience, this raises the question of how, if at all, they are equipped to change the *status quo*. This can be seen in the relationship between the patient and doctor or other health worker in which, predictably, the patient grants authority to the doctor, acknowledging the power of the doctor and their subordinate status. This establishes the parameters of the relationship and enhances the opportunity to achieve their collective objectives. It also reduces the need for, and use of, threats or incentives. These are replaced by a mutual understanding of the relationship itself, and the consequences of operating outside the agreed parameters (the advice and prescription for care offered by the doctor). Patients are influenced because they want to follow and sustain their motivation by either recognition that their symptoms are subsiding, or justifying their subordinate behaviour in this relationship for the overall goal of getting well.

Power and leadership

Stogdill (1948) suggested that leadership may be considered as the process or act of, influencing the activities of an organised group, in its efforts toward goal setting and goal achievement. Bryman (1986) considered leadership from a more conceptual basis and proposed that the concept leadership involves, 'the creation of a vision about a desired future state which seeks to enmesh all members of an organisation in its net'.

The common themes within these definitions imply that leadership involves a degree of social influence in which one person guides members of a group (followers) towards their goal. When we apply these ideas to health care and place the service user in the role of the follower, the behaviour and actions of the professional gain significant emphasis. Collinson (1995) suggested that doctors are the élite and have a special relationship with their patients, are highly selected and represent some of the best people of their generation, undergoing long and demanding training. He concludes that all the numerous sociological studies show doctors to be at the apex of society's status pyramid. Yet the characteristics set out here are the very antithesis of what many experience when attempting to negotiate successfully health and welfare systems. The genius of a leader is to articulate a vision, simple enough to be understood, appealing enough to evoke commitment, and credible enough to be accepted as realistic and attainable (Yuki, 1989). Visionary leaders have the ability to hypothesise and construct scenarios from the presenting situation. They must combine experience, personality, abstract thinking, foresight and 'gut feeling' to produce the vision (*Figure 1.1*).

The trait approach

This approach subscribes to the view that leaders are born not made, and stems from research undertaken in the 1940s (Bird, 1940; Stogdill, 1948).

No amount of learning will make a man a leader unless he has the natural qualities of one (General Archibald Wavell, 1941) (*Table 1.1*).

Some characteristics of a leader	Some characteristics of a follower
Good listener	Good talker
Accessible	Hard to find
Decisive	Avoids decisions
Straightforward	Makes it complicated
Optimistic	Pessimistic
Gives credit	Always takes credit
Confronts problems	Avoids problems
Speaks directly	Manipulates
Acknowledges mistakes	Blames others
Says yes	Explains why it cannot be done
Able to say no	Cannot say no
Enthusiastic	Placid or cynical
Seeks strong subordinates	Seeks weak subordinates
Positive attitude	Negative attitude

Figure 1.1: Characteristics of leaders and followers

Table 1.1: Desirable leadership traits

Physical characteristics	Social background	Intelligence and ability
Active, energetic	Educated	Judgement
Smart, well-groomed	Social status	Decisive
	Mobility	Knowledgeable
		Articulate

Personality	Task-related characteristics	Social characteristics
Adaptable	Achievement, drive, desire to excel	Ability to enlist cooperation
Aggressive	Shows initiative	Administrative ability
Assertive	Has a desire for responsibility	Ability to cooperate
Dominant	Task oriented	Popular
Emotionally balanced	Persists against obstacles	Sociable
Independent		Good interpersonal skills
Objective		Tact, diplomacy
Creative		
Moral		
Trustworthy		
Self-confident		
Has strength of conviction		
Able to cope with stress		

Based on: Bass' (1981) interpretation of Stodgill's research (1948, 1970)

The style approach

In the late 1940s, the study of leadership shifted away from its emphasis on traits and personal characteristics to that of the leader's style and behaviour.

A move from what the leader 'has' to what the leader 'does'.

Many writers have attempted to classify leadership styles, with the majority falling along the autocratic democratic continuum.

Autocratic _ Democratic

Research has emphasised two main areas of behaviour, which is associated with leadership (Bryman, 1989):

- consideration
- initiating structure.

A considerate leader is one who has a relationship of trust with subordinates and respects their views and feelings.

A leader who exhibits a high degree of structuring is one who attempts to define and structure the work of subordinates.

Leaders who are considerate tend to be liked by their subordinates, but are often considered less effective by their own leaders/managers. In contrast, their subordinates mostly dislike leaders who exhibit initiating structures. This suggests that there may be tension between these two styles:

Autocratic	Democratic	Consultative	Laissez-faire

When comparing autocratic and democratic styles of leadership, the issue of power must be considered.

An autocratic leader holds the balance if not all of the power, whereas a democratic leader shares the power with the group.

There is a general assumption that people will be more productive working in a democratic regime rather than an authoritarian regime. Is this the case?

Arguments for this idea promote the notion that increased participation in the decision-making process satisfies the self-actualisation and esteem needs of the individual, leading to a more productive worker. Another idea is that participation affects one's need for stimulation and variety of work, leading to a more productive worker. Handy (1993) pointed out that this creates an atmosphere where:

- workers may feel more satisfied
- there is a lower staff turnover and grievance rate
- there is less inter-group conflict
- subordinates are happier.

The contingency approach

The notion that overall effectiveness cannot rely on either style or traits alone has led to the emergence of the contingency approach. The central focus of this argument is that particular styles, behaviours and traits are only appropriate in particular circumstances.

Supporters of this theory focus on the variables involved in the leadership situation.

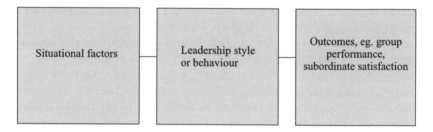

Figure 1.2: Fielder's theory, 1967

Fielder concentrated upon the relationship between the leader and the group, and the structure of the task as determinants in the most effective style of leadership.

He used the term psychologically distant, and psychologically close, and proposed that effective leaders maintain a greater psychological distance between themselves and their subordinates. His research demonstrated that:

❖ The psychologically distant leader tended to be role orientated in interactions with both subordinates and superiors.

❖ The psychologically distant leader held regular formal meetings.

❖ The psychologically distant leader demanded and received considerable freedom from their superiors.

For the psychologically distant leader to be effective they must be informally accepted by the group, and if this condition is not met the group 'will not listen to him'.

The task must be clearly defined and the group's respect must be high and the leader could reward or punish the subordinates. In contrast:

❖ The psychologically close leader saw his job as primarily ensuring smooth interpersonal relations with everyone.

❖ The psychologically close leader tended to develop close personal ties with people.

❖ The psychologically close leader held few formal meetings.

Fielder concluded that the psychologically close leader generally felt the need to dominate and possess others, and achieves less in terms of productivity.

The transformational approach

The concept of the transformational leader was coined by Burns (1978) who described this person as one who:

- empowers
- has a long-term focus
- challenges
- rewards informally
- is emotional
- mixes home and work
- inspires through vision and ideals
- is able to simplify and translate complex ideas.

The transformational leader is said to be able to inspire others to greater achievement, enhancing motivation and involvement in the leader's cause.

This was contrasted with the transactional leader who relies on followers being induced to comply through an incentive, ie. money, status, etc. This 'rarely binds the leader and follower together in a mutual and common pursuit of a higher purpose' (Burns, 1978).

Political power and a meritocratic society

The essence of a meritocratic society is that it offers individuals an equal opportunity to become unequal (Saunders, 1996). The competitive nature of such a society produces both winners and losers where the most desirable reward and highest status positions are attained by the most successful and talented. This supports the notion that social position and power is gained through the application of talent and hard work, rather than through inherited or birthright social position and power.

Pluralism is a term often used as a defence of what might otherwise be called liberal democracy or representative or participatory democracy. A pluralist political system is one that seems to be a development from elitism, and has several centres of power and authority, rather than one where the state is the sole controller of people's actions. For example, trade unions and industrial associations, along with political parties and perhaps the administrative bureaucracy, effectively share power with the official government and legislature. This is in contrast to an oligarchy where groups are ruled by a few and the larger the group, the more concentrated the power (Michels, 1967).

One version of pluralist theory has come to be known as a polyarchy, where interest groups and pressure groups exist in relatively stable tension with each other. This forms the basis of power in most Western societies.

The voluntary sector in health care has developed in tandem with the NHS. Whelan (1999) suggested that throughout the 1980s and 1990s governments have struggled with the seemingly intractable problem of rising public demand for high quality welfare services, coupled with an unwillingness to pay taxes for them. In answer, politicians have rediscovered the virtues of volunteerism. Voluntary organisations, pressure groups and those concerned with advocacy fall into three categories:

- those who rely on charitable status
- those who are the paid employees of the organisations they are set to challenge
- those who are funded directly or indirectly from Government.

There is perhaps a fourth group, those who rely on a combination of these methods for funding, but essentially each model is flawed. Organisations who rely on their charitable status, perpetuate under-funding by the government by filling in gaps in provision that should be provided by statutory services. Individuals and organisations who are in the paid employment of their mother organisation, have a vested interest in sustaining their source of funding and therefore may acquiesce to the will of their employer to 'loose the battle for the sake of the war'. This system can never offer the independence required to be able to represent or advocate effectively. Those who are funded directly or indirectly from Government, for example, Community Health Councils in 1974 effectively institutionalised the voice of the community within the NHS (Klein and Lewis, 1976).

Structural functionalists see professional power as a static and secure social stratum, which provides a socially cohesive role to stabilise the forces that may fragment society (Parsons, 1939; Goode, 1957). They are said to conform to a set pattern of predictable traits and events and from a Weberian perspective undertake strategies to promote their own social status (Freidson, 1970; Saks, 1983). This self-serving approach is designed to persuade potential customers of a need for their service. It also has the effect of ring-fencing that service, and ensuring that it is provided exclusively by those within the professional group. In this case, power can be seen as being closely connected to one's social identity and as Foucault (1980) proposes, being a means of legitimating dominance of one group over another.

Pilgrim and Rogers (1999) suggested that professionals exercise power over others in three senses. Firstly, they do this by convincing clients that they have a specialised knowledge and thus keeping their customer or client in a state of ignorance, insecurity and vulnerability. Secondly, they create a hierarchy in which those who wish to join their ranks must endure initiation (perhaps through a form of particular training) and commence at the bottom of the ladder. Thirdly, professional groups continually vie with each other for dominance over each other if working with a similar client group or customer base. This can be seen clearly in the efforts of the nursing profession to aspire academically and develop a conceptual and evidence base from which to compete for dominance with their medical colleagues. The abject failure of *Project 2000* (UKCC, 1986) gives testimony to the fact that the essence of nursing is a pragmatic, task-orientated and subordinate role to medicine. Post *Project 2000* curricula emphasise the unique nature of that task, thereby re-establishing the distinctive role nurses play in health care, and implicitly acknowledging the failure to persuade themselves and other professions of professional equity. It could be said that the desire of the nursing profession to be seen as equitable to medicine was merely an opportunistic attempt to capitalise on a growing weakness and capture the public mood. As patients, we are increasingly sceptical and argumentative, and few of us are still prepared to regard the doctor as god (Cardy *et al*, 1999). Nursing is not the only profession to attempt to unseat medicine from its dominant position. Flying the flag for psychology, Pilgrim (2000) suggests that:

> *Diagnosis is a medical task that creates a simple dichotomy between the sick and the well, in contrast, psychological formulations assume a continuity between the normal and the abnormal.*

Key points

- ⌘ If power is the ability to achieve or promote the interests one holds, then the powerful health professional will acknowledge the need for partnership, and strive to share elements of their role in which the recipient of care may contribute. Rather than detract from their power base, it will enhance it, as a concordant relationship will produce a more sustainable health gain than one based upon compliance.
- ⌘ Professionals must engage survivors to redress imbalances in the power relationship, learn from real experiences, and recognise that the discomfort and tension produced by the process will be offset by the rewards for all concerned.
- ⌘ Empowerment will emanate from good leadership, combining experience, personality, abstract thinking, foresight and gut feeling to produce the creativity necessary to translate the vision into action.
- ⌘ A state of 'defused tension' is an outcome of empowerment which recognises the potential for destructive power, and uses this to enable progressive change.
- ⌘ If empowerment of service users is to occur, it must have organisational support and cannot rely upon a single individual.

References

Bass BM (1981) *Stodgill's Handbook of Leadership*. Free Press, New York: 375–6

Beveridge W (1948) *Voluntary Action: A report on the methods of social advance*. George Allen & Unwin, London

Bird C (1940) *Social Psychology*. Appleton-Century, New York

Brooker C, Repper J, eds. (1998) *Serious Mental Health Problems in the Community: Policy practice and research*. Baillière Tindall, London

Bryman A (1986) *Leadership and Organisations*. Routledge and Kegan Paul, London: 6

Bryman A (1989) Leadership and culture in organisations. *Public Money and Management*, Autumn: 429–36

Burns JM (1978) *Leadership*. Harper and Rowe, New York: 224

Cardy P, Cayton H, Edwards B, Gay H (1999) *Keeping Patients in the Dark: Should prescription medicines be advertised direct to the consumers?* Institute of Economic Affairs, London: 22

Collinson P (1995) *Patients or Customers: Are the NHS Reforms Working?* Institute of Economic Affairs, London

Department of Health (1971) *Better Services for the Mentally Handicapped*. Cmnd 4683. HMSO, London

Department of Health (1975) *Better Services for the Mentally Ill*. Cmnd 6233. HMSO, London

Department of Health (1989) *Caring for People: Community care in the next decade and beyond*. Cmnd 849. HMSO, London

Department of Health (1991) *The Patients' Charter*. London. DoH, London

Department of Health (2001) *Your guide to the NHS*. Online at http://www.nhs.uk/nhsguide

Dooher J, Byrt R, eds (2002) *Empowerment and the Health Service User*. Quay Books, Mark Allen Publishing Ltd, Dinton, Wiltshire

Fielder FE (1967) *A Theory of Leadership Effectiveness*. McGraw Hill, New York

Foucault M (1980) *Power/Knowledge: Selected interviews and other writings 1972–1977*. Harvester Wheatsheaf, New York: 119

Freidson E (1970) *Profession of Medicine*. Harper and Row, New York

French JP, Raven B (1959) *The Bases of Social Power in Studies in Social Power*. Cartwright D, ed. Institute for Social Research, London: 150–67

Goffman E (1961) *Asylums: Essays on the social situation of mental patients and other inmates*. Penguin Books, Harmondsworth

Goode W (1957) Community within a community: the professions. *Am Sociological Rev* **xx**(1): 194–200

Handy C (1993) *Understanding Organisations*. Penguin, London: 100

Klein R, Lewis J (1976) *The Politics of Consumer Representation*. Centre for Studies in Social Policy, London

Lindow V (1990) Participation and power. *Open MIND* **44**: 10

Lindow V (1991) Experts, lies and stereotypes. *Health Serv J* **101**(5267): 18–9

Michels R (1967) *Political Parties*. Free Press, New York

Parsons T (1939) The professions and the social structure. *Social Forces* **17**: 457–67

Parsons T (1957) Illness and the role of the physician: a sociological perspective. *Am J Orthopsychiatry*. **2**: 452 – 460. In: Hamilton P, ed. *Readings from Talcott Parsons*. Open University Press, Milton Keynes

Pembroke L (1991) Surviving psychiatry. *Nurs Times* **87**(49): 30–2

Pilgrim D, Rogers A (1999) *A Sociology of Mental Health and Illness*. 2nd edn. Milton Keynes. Open University Press, Milton Keynes

Pilgrim D (2000) Psychiatric diagnosis: More questions than answers. *Psychologist* **13**(6): 302–4

Saks M (1983) Removing the blinkers? A critique of recent contributions to the sociology of professions. *Sociological Rev* **33**: 1–22

Saunders P (1996) *Unequal but Fair? A study of class barriers in Britain*. Institute of Economic Affairs, London: 76

Seligman MEP (1973) *Helplessness. On depression, development and death*. Freeman, San Francisco

Stogdill RM, Shartle CL (1948) Methods for determining patterns of leadership behaviour in relation to organisation structure and objectives. *J Appl Psychol* **32**: 286–91

United Kingdom Central Council for Nursing, Midwifery and Health Visiting (1999) *Fitness for practice and purpose*. UKCC, London

United Kingdom Central Council for Nursing, Midwifery and Health Visiting (1986) *Project 2000. A New Preparation for Practice*. UKCCC, London

Wavell, General A (1941) The Art of Generalship. *The Times*, 17 February, 1941. Cited in: Bryman A (1986) *Leadership and Organisations*. Routledge and Keegan Paul, London: 18

Whelan R (1999) *Involuntary Action: How voluntary is the voluntary sector?* Institute of Economic Affairs, London: 15

Yuki GA (1989) *Leadership in Organisations*. Prentice Hall, Englewood Cliffs, NJ: 120

2

Empowerment and participation: definitions, meanings and models

Richard Byrt and James Dooher

... Inherent in [many] arguments is the underlying assumption that empowerment is... a 'good thing', and that by acting in an empowering way, health professionals will become more effective and patients will become healthier...

(Kendall, 1998b, p. 1)

... The concept of participation has been widely recognised by many health care professionals to be a good thing... [but] there is an urgent call for hard evidence to show that patient participation is of value to the patient and the clinician...

(Cahill, 1998, p. 126)

Several authors have noted that both 'empowerment' and 'participation' are 'value words', seen by many proponents as good in themselves, with, in some cases, enthusiastic and uncritical acceptance. As long ago as 1969, Arnstein commented of participation:

Everyone is for participation... it can't be bad. But who is able to say what it is?

(Arnstein, 1969, p. 216)

This chapter considers some definitions and explores the meanings of empowerment, participation and related concepts. The term 'service user' will be used throughout to refer to clients and patients of health services, including people who receive care and treatment reluctantly or against their will. The term 'carer' is used to indicate an individual who provides informal or unpaid care for someone, usually in their own home. The authors are aware that some people so described object to, or have not chosen, these terms. However, they are used in the absence of apparent universally agreed alternatives, and because of their widespread use in the literature. (For a discussion of related issues, see Chapter 1 in the companion volume to this book, Dooher and Byrt, 2002a.)

Empowerment: definitions

Much of the literature on empowerment includes observations that this term lacks clear definition and conceptualisation (Skelton, 1994; Gale, 1998; Kuokkannen and Leino-Kilpi, 2000) and is used imprecisely in some of the literature. Gale (1998) comments that empowerment is 'a nebulous term' and Skelton (1994) states that definitions are 'varied and imprecise'. Barnes and Bowl (2001) refer to the wide range of ways in which the term has been used within health and social services and community development. McLean argues that the concept of empowerment has been:

> *... diluted ... distorted ... [and] has assumed diverse and even contradictory meanings ... It may refer to a process, a goal to be achieved, or a combination of these.*
>
> (McLean 1995, quoted in Jackson, 1997, p. 50; and Jackson and Hislop, 2002)

Empowerment has been said to be difficult to implement or put into practice (Gale, 1998; Kendall, 1998b; Laverack and Wallerstein, 2001) and difficult to measure (Gibson, 1995; Laverack and Wallerstein, 2001). Kendall comments that:

> *... there are very few analyses of the way in which the process of empowerment can be practised or the outcome of empowerment identified...*
>
> (Kendall 1998b, p. 1)

Tones (1998a) states:

> *... if programmes designed to empower are effectively designed and their effectiveness is to be demonstrated, the concept of empowerment must be operationalised and its implications opened up to scrutiny...*
>
> (Tones 1998a, p. 185)

The implementation and measurement of both empowerment and participation can be facilitated by identifying their components or constituent parts, and their dimensions, including degrees and levels, ie. the amount and extent of empowerment and participation. In relation to the dimensions of empowerment, many definitions of the concept refer to one, two or more of the following:

Dimensions of empowerment

❖ Psychological or individual: The individual service user's/carer's feelings of power and/or control related to factors such as his/her skills, aptitudes and abilities, confidence, self-efficacy (belief in the capacity to bring about change, Tones, 1998a), self-worth and pride in identity.

❖ Service-initiated: Professionals and managers enabling service users and carers to gain and/or share power.

❖ Service change: The successful bringing about of change desired by the service user/carer, usually with his/her active participation.

❖ Social inclusion and social change: This includes access to the quality of life and life opportunities enjoyed by most people, elimination of discrimination and stigmatisation; and the gaining of political power.

Some definitions focus on only one of these dimensions. For example, empowerment has been defined as, 'a process of helping people to assert control over the factors that affect their lives' (Fraher and Limpinnian, 1999, p. 146, citing Gibson, 1991). Kendall (1998b) stated that the 'World Health Organization's definition of health promotion' is often used as a basis for definitions of empowerment: '... the process of enabling people to increase control over, and to improve their health' (Kendall, 1998b, p.2, quoting the World Health Organization, 1986). Braye and Preston–Shoot (1995) commented that, when based on traditional values, empowerment involves:

> *... enabling people to acquire the skills and confidence needed to bring about improvements in the quality of their lives, or helping people to compete more effectively for scarce resources...*

> (Braye and Preston-Shoot,1995, p. 50)

A definition proposed by Rodwell (1996) included a number of dimensions of empowerment:

> *... the process of enabling or imparting power transfer from an individual or group to another. It includes the elements of power, authority, choice and permission...*

> *... It is a process of enabling people to choose to take control over and make decisions about their lives. It is also a process which values all those involved...*

However, Kendall (1998b) concluded that empowerment, 'is not a simple transfer of power from one individual to another' (p. 3), a point considered below. Kendall referred to a definition of Gibson:

Empowerment is a social process of recognition, promoting and enhancing people's abilities to meet their own needs, solve their own problems and mobilise the necessary resources in order to feel in control of their own lives...

(Kendall, 1998b, p. 3, quoting Gibson, 1991, p. 359)

Parsloe (1996) argued that it would be difficult to offer a 'definitive definition of empowerment... because the concept is still evolving and means different things to different people' (Parsloe, 1996, quoted in Barnes and Bowl, 2001, p. 18). Nevertheless, her consideration of its meaning also covers a number of dimensions:

Empowerment... is used to refer to users of social services having greater control over the services they receive and is here concerned with the individual service level. It can also refer to a more general level of planning for services at the local, regional or national level when service users are involved in advising, and less frequently, in deciding on the services to be provided. It may be seen as a way to reduce professional power or a plot used cynically by professionals to protect their status and power. Its purpose may be to promote the quality and appropriateness of social services or to give disadvantaged members of society some influence which may lead to their attaining greater political power.

(Parsloe, 1996, quoted in
Barnes and Bowl, 2001, p. 18)

Dimensions and types of empowerment in the literature

A number of authors have distinguished between various dimensions and types of empowerment. In their review of community participation in community health promotion, Bracht *et al* (1999) distinguish between psychological (sometimes called individual) empowerment and community empowerment:

Psychological empowerment can be defined as a subjective feeling of greater control over one's life that an individual experiences following active membership in groups or organisations...

(Bracht *et al*, 1999, p. 86)

These authors go on to state that community empowerment is 'participation in collective political action' which can result in both increased psychological empowerment and, '... the achievement of some redistribution of resources or decision making sought by a community or sub-group' (Bracht *et al*, 1999, p. 87). Rogers *et al* (1997, cited in Barnes and Bowl, 2001, p. 18) developed measures of both 'psychological and political dimensions of empowerment' (see *p. 26*). *Chapter 5* considers further the links between empowerment at psychological (individual) and community levels (see also, Green and Tones, 2002).

Some critics have argued that psychological empowerment does not necessarily lead to redistributions of power or desired outcomes, eg. changes in the provision of health services. Tones pointed out that:

People's health is not just an individual responsibility. Our health is to a large extent governed by the physical, social, cultural and economic environments in which we live and work...

(Tones 1998b, p. 59)

The Health of the Nation (DoH, 1992) was criticised for failing to take social and political factors into account in setting targets to improve health. The document appeared to be based on assumptions that factors associated, for instance, with coronary heart disease and suicide, were solely related to the individual. In contrast, *Saving Lives. Our Healthier Nation* (DoH, 1998b) considered some of the social and political factors which impinge on health (Fatchett, 1998). Melluish (1998) refers to the work of Smail, who argued that:

... power is not solely a psychological phenomenon... but is linked to 'coercive economic and ideological factors'. This conceptualisation of power implies that 'empowerment' can only take place where there is a shift in such resources towards those in less powerful positions...

(Melluish, 1998, p. 264f, quoting Smail, 1994)

Kuokkanen and Leino-Kilpi (2000, p. 238) stated that writing on empowerment is based on three groups of theories:

* Critical social theory, which is concerned with devolving power to oppressed groups: eg. many health service clients, including those who are women, members of minority ethnic groups or who have disabilities or are lesbian or gay.
* Organisational and management theories, which stress the benefits of empowerment to both the individual and the organisation as a whole.
* Social psychological theories, in which 'empowerment' is seen as a process of personal growth and development.

Development of empowerment in the individual

Some research suggests that both empowerment and participation develop incrementally, in a number of stages, which may be related to increases in the individual's knowledge, confidence and self-efficacy: components of psychological or individual empowerment (Byrt and Dooher, 2002; Gibson, 1995; Tones, 1998a; Tones, 1998b). Gibson described five stages towards empowerment in mothers of children with long-term neurological illnesses. These included:

1. Discovering reality, including seeking information about their child's condition.
2. Frustration, partly related to delays in appointments and professionals' dismissal of problems.
3. Critical reflection, in which mothers evaluated situations, developed confidence and took positive action.
4. Taking charge, including:
   * 'advocating for the child'
   * 'dealing effectively with the hospital system'
   * 'learning to persist'
   * negotiation with professionals
   * establishing partnerships with professionals.
5. Holding on: the development of personal control, even in crises, with the discovery of meaning and a 'sense of purpose' (Gibson, 1995, p. 79).

In contrast to findings that information and knowledge enable, or are an important component of empowerment (Coulter *et al*, 1998), most research on individuals living with diabetes has found that, 'levels of knowledge decrease with age, and also with the duration of the disease, which is surprising, considering chronic illness theories of learning to cope with the disease over periods of time' (Gillibrand and Flynn, 2001, p. 503). Postulated reasons for this apparent diminution of knowledge include service users' high levels of anxiety when they first receive education from professionals, and the latter's lack of competence in giving explanations (Gillibrand and Flynn, 2001). A failure to consider seriously service users' perspectives, recognise and respect their own knowledge, or adapt information and advice to their life circumstances may also be important (Paterson, 2001). This disregard for service users' knowledge may be related to the relatively dominant power of professional discourses (Miers, 1999). (Discourse has been defined as, '... commonly accepted assumptions that claim to explain reality and therefore form a base for knowledge', Wilkinson, 1999, p. 21, citing Foucault, 1980. See also *Chapter 3* and Godfrey, 2002.)

Components of empowerment

An appreciation of the complexity of the concept of empowerment, and of its many components or constituent parts, appears to be essential in the effective implementation of care and services to increase empowerment. Components of empowerment frequently identified in the literature (eg. Hogg, 1999; Kemshall and Littlechild, 2000; Kendall, 1998a; Wilkinson and Miers, 1999) are listed in *Figure 2.1*, in relation to specific dimensions. These components are considered in other parts of this book.

Components of empowerment overlap with those of participation. In addition, some of the identified components themselves facilitate empowerment and participation. For example, high self-efficacy and self-esteem are likely to facilitate an individual's choices regarding his/her care and participating in attempts to change services, increase political power or decrease social exclusion. Equally, components of psychological or individual empowerment may be facilitated (or hindered) by professionals' communication styles and treatment models, as well as by service users'/carers' power to bring about changes in services and in the wider community, eg. in relation to increased life opportunities (Bracht *et al*, 1999). Factors facilitating empowerment and participation are considered in Dooher and Byrt (2002b) in the companion volume to this book.

Dimension	Components
Individual or psychological Client's belief and ability to have power, influence or control	• awareness of oppression • consciousness raising • pride in identity • increase in self-esteem • increased internal locus of control • increased self-efficacy
Service-initiated Professionals'/managers' willingness to empower service users/carers in individual care, service delivery, health policies and wider society	• professional-service user/carer communication and relationships • professional attitudes • professional cultures, discourses and treatment models • organisational cultures and structures • systems to enable empowerment and participation
Service change Service users'/carers' **actual** achievement of change, power or control over individual care, wider service provision or policy	• consultation • information • choice • having a voice • availability and accessibility of services • autonomy • participation in decision making • control • influence • rights/advocacy • power
Social inclusion and social change Achievement of social inclusion involving social and political changes, equality of opportunity and freedom from discrimination in wider society	• full citizenship and rights • equality In relation to: • life opportunities, choices and control (eg. related to privacy, independence, relationships, accommodation and meaningful activity) • quality of life • freedom from discrimination stereotyping and other negative attitudes • putting forward alternative discourses which challenge existing power imbalances • political power

Figure 2.1: Dimensions of empowerment

Chamberlin (1997) and Barnes and Bowl (2001) produce particularly comprehensive lists of components of empowerment. Barnes and Bowl (2001, p. 24) include items concerned with all the dimensions identified. Their list includes:

- 'personal growth and development'
- improving health
- influence in relation to services received by the individual and others
- changes within families and other social groups
- increased 'control over life choices'
- 'resistance to and subversion of dominant discourses and practices' and the development by service users and carers of valued alternative 'knowledges'
- translating ideas about empowerment into action
- gaining 'a presence in political systems from which you have been excluded'
- achieving 'structural change'
- 'reducing inequalities'.

Measures of empowerment and the need to consider all four dimensions

Byrt and Dooher suggest that in relation to health service users and carers:

❖ General definitions and models of empowerment are not complete unless they consider all four of the dimensions identified in *Figure 2.1*.

❖ Maximum empowerment exists when the individual is empowered in relation to all four dimensions. This can be expressed as:

$$A + B + C + D = E$$

where A, B, C and D are psychological (individual), service-initiated, service change and social inclusion/social change dimensions, respectively; and E represents maximum opportunities for service user or carer empowerment.

Researchers have evaluated the extent that certain dimensions of empowerment exist (Kendall, 1998a); and in some cases, have used the research process itself as a means to empower service users and carers (Kemshall and Littlechild, 2000.) However, the authors are unaware of research that has assessed the total amount of empowerment experienced by service users or carers on all four dimensions. In relation to the latter, perhaps a total score could be estimated, using the above formula, to indicate the extent that an individual is empowered. The meaning and meaningfulness of such a measure, particularly to service users/carers, as well as issues of reliability and validity, would, of course, need to be considered carefully (Cormack, 2000). Furthermore, it has been argued that it is difficult to produce a 'universal measure' of empowerment because 'it may not mean the same thing for every person, organisation, or community everywhere' (Laverack and Wallerstein, 2001, p. 182). In addition, some aspects of empowerment (particularly those related to the social change/social inclusion dimension) are dynamic and changing, with individuals experiencing varying amounts of empowerment at different times and in relation to different situations (Laverack and Wallerstein, 2001).

There has been an increasing amount of research on a variety of aspects of psychological and service-initiated empowerment (*Chapter 5*; Faulkner, 2001; Leskell *et al*, 2001; Paterson, 2001). Some measures of quality of life have included items of relevance to social inclusion (Draper, 1997; Priestley, 1999). Public and professional attitude scales, including measures of stigmatisation of particular groups of individuals, are also of relevance (Mason *et al*, 2001). Rogers *et al* (1997) produced a scale to measure several dimensions of empowerment:

> *Self-efficacy-self-esteem, power-powerlessness, community activism, righteous anger, and optimism — control over the future. These criteria reflect both psychological and political dimensions of the concept.*

> (Barnes and Bowl, 2001, p. 18,
> citing Rogers *et al*, 1997)

Laverack and Wallerstein (2001) reviewed the difficulties in measuring and implementing empowerment in local communities. In order to promote this, these authors proposed better conceptual understanding of empowerment, community participation in the development of methodologies and planned action, based on information collected. Laverack and Wallerstein also referred to the importance, in relation to effective measurement, of distinguishing between process, involving psychological empowerment, and outcome in relation to effecting political and social change.

An individual service user or carer can experience varying amounts of empowerment across these and other dimensions. Professionals in a primary healthcare team may endeavour to empower a service user, and through community health projects, reduce social exclusion. Despite these efforts, he/she may have low self-esteem and low self-efficacy. Conversely, a highly motivated individual, who is prepared to persevere in the face of difficulties, might have a high degree of individual empowerment, despite disempowering professional attitudes and relationships and unsuccessful attempts to influence service provision.

Empowerment within each dimension

In addition, within each dimension, there may be empowerment in some ways, but not in others, as illustrated in the examples below.

Psychological or individual dimension

Alan Amber, who is living with AIDS, has high self-esteem and a positive self-identity, with a refusal to internalise others' stigmatising attitudes. However, he has low self-efficacy, feeling unable to believe that any action he takes will influence either his own health or service provision for other people living with AIDS. Indeed, Mr Amber does not expect to have such influence. (This example perhaps calls into question the extent that low self-efficacy can co-exist with high self-esteem; see *Chapter 5*.)

Service-initiated dimension

Managers working in a medical unit in a general hospital make themselves accessible to local carers, who are concerned about the care their elderly relatives and partners receive in the hospital. There is great interest in the views of the carers, and recommendations are made, following a management-initiated survey of their views. However, managers lack the ability to implement the recommendations in order to bring about change, or to change the organisational cultures of wards in order to do so. The style of leadership is likely to be important here (*Chapter 1*), as is the willingness of different participants to share power.

Service change dimension

A voluntary organisation of individuals with learning disabilities and their carers and other advocates campaign to have opportunities to influence central Government policies related to the services provided. They are delighted to find that their lobbying has influenced decisions to ensure that they participate in a Government planning forum for these services. However, after three years, they feel disillusioned as their views have had little practical effect on service delivery. Not only is the policy and opportunity for individuals to participate relevant here, but their power and influence to achieve desired change. (Barnes and Bowl [2001] refer to the resignation of service users from a DoH national group on mental health, after they were unable to influence policy designed to ensure compliance with medication in the community.)

Social inclusion and social change dimension

Empowerment and participation of people who are service users and carers may have limited benefit if they are seen only in terms of these roles, and suffer social exclusion (Sayce, 2000). After years of lobbying the local council, Barbara Beige and other members of a group campaigning for independent living have gained funding to employ their own personal assistants. Ms Beige has found that this has enabled her to engage in a much wider range of activities in her local town, although the arrangement is not as flexible as she would like it to be. Moreover, her access to the range of nightclubs that she can attend is constrained by lack of wheelchair access and the patronising attitudes of some of the other clubbers and staff (this example draws on Priestley, 1999).

The relationship of these dimensions of empowerment to participation is considered briefly at the end of this chapter. The next part of this chapter considers participation.

Participation: definitions

Several authors note the wide range of meanings attributed to participation, and the lack of agreement about the definition of the concept. Cahill comments that the term, '... is widely used in the literature to describe various approaches to health care'; and refers to a 'distinct lack of consensus concerning the meaning of patient participation' (Cahill, 1998, p. 44).

Dictionary definitions of participation include the following:

to take part in, to become actively involved in, to share in...

(Smithies and Webster, 1998, p. 84,
quoting *Collins English Dictionary*)

The 'Shorter Oxford English Dictionary' gives at least two definitions: one implies the idea of forming part of something, the second that of sharing something in common with others, or taking part with others, in some action or other.

(Boaden *et al*, 1982, p. 11, citing the
Shorter Oxford English Dictionary)

Boaden *et al* (1982) stated that these dictionary definitions raise further questions about the meaning of 'taking part', and the precise nature of participation, and consideration of which people are the participants.

In the literature, definitions of participation include the idea of individuals taking part, or being actively involved, in an activity or in a service that they receive. Byrt (1994) found a lack of definitions of service user/carer participation in the literature, and proposed the following definition:

... the involvement of [service users/carers] in responsibility and/or decision making, which has an intended impact on services and/or policies which affect the individual participant and/or other [service users/carers].

(Byrt, 1994, p. 49)

Cahill (1998) quoted a definition of Brownlea (1987), who stated that participation means:

... getting involved, or being allowed to become involved, in the decision making process or the delivery of a service, or even simply to become one of a number of people consulted on an issue or matter.

(Cahill, 1998, p. 120, quoting Brownlea, 1987)

Cahill (1998) commented that most definitions fail to indicate the complexity of participation:

> *In a multi-national survey considered by Kim et al (1993) it was found that cultural heritage, social development and country of residence were all major structural variables that contributed to different patient and practitioner views about the nature of the phenomenon and how it is executed in practice.*

(Cahill, 1998, p. 120)

Various terms such as 'involvement', 'partnership' and 'collaboration', in relation to health service users, are often used interchangeably with 'participation' (Byrt, 1994; Cahill, 1998, Smithies and Webster, 1998.) However, professional – client partnerships have been considered as a distinct concept (Coulter, 1997; Florin and Coulter, 2001); and collaboration and involvement as a component of both participation and empowerment (Shemmings and Shemmings, 1995). According to Shaw (2000), the term 'user involvement' is strongly associated with consumerism: the introduction of market principles into public services, with measurements of client satisfaction and systems for investigating complaints. Shaw (2000) adds that 'participation' is more likely to be associated with involvement in decision making, and responsibility in important aspects of service provision and planning. A similar distinction has been made between democratic and consumerist participation. In the former, empowerment is seen as resulting from political initiatives in order to develop state welfare, equitable income distribution and citizens' rights. Service users and carers are involved in major policy making and management of services (Braye, 2000; Lupton *et al*, 1998). Consumer participation is concerned with high standards of 'information, access, choice and redress' (Lupton *et al*, 1998, p. 50) and other aspects of service quality (Braye, 2000). There is an emphasis on service users'/ carers' views about quality issues in consumer approaches, and this may inform decision making (Byrt, 2001).

Dimensions of participation

From research on participation, conducted in the mid-1980s, and a review of the literature, Byrt (1994) concluded that the complexity of participation could be understood through the consideration of eight dimensions (Byrt, 1994; McFadyen and Farrington, 1997). These dimensions, represented in *Figure 2.2*, comprise:

- degrees
- levels
- components, types and methods
- modes of intervention
- types of participant
- openness
- consciousness
- formality.

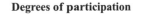
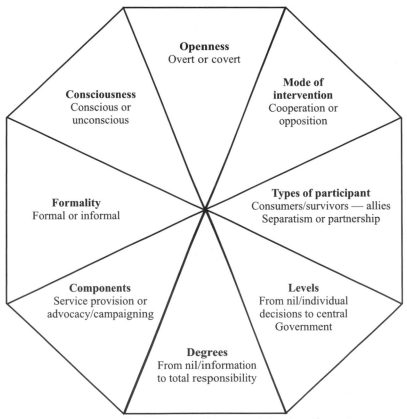

Figure 2.2: Octagon of service user/carer participation (from Byrt, 1994 and McFadyen and Farrington, 1997)

Some of these dimensions can also be used to understand the nature of empowerment. Each of these will now be considered in turn, except for 'types of participant', a topic considered in Byrt and Dooher (2002) (in the companion volume to this book) and 'types and methods', which are covered in many of the subsequent chapters.

Degrees of participation, empowerment and power

Degrees of participation refer to varying amounts of involvement, from 'no participation' to 'total control of the organisation'. A number of typologies of degrees of participation have been devised, including those differentiating between 'true participation' and what has variously been described as 'false participation', 'pseudo-participation' and 'tokenism'. The latter terms refer to apparent 'participation', imposed or granted by people in positions of power, who have already made the decisions (Midgley *et al*, 1986; Shemmings and Shemmings, 1995). Several authors refer to 'tokenism' as giving 'participation' to an individual as a gesture, without allowing or enabling him/her to have the power to make a difference (Chamberlin, 1988). Shiffman (2002) described an Indonesian family planning project which, although seen as a shining example of community empowerment in practice, was largely controlled at various stages by central government, with limited opportunities for public participation. However, as Kennedy (2001) has outlined, meaningful community participation is sometimes difficult to implement.

An early typology of participation is Arnstein's Ladder (Arnstein, 1969), which has since been adapted by other authors (Braye, 2000; Shemmings and Shemmings, 1995). In Arnstein's Ladder, the lowest two rungs, 'manipulation' and 'therapy' were classed as non-participation; and rungs three to five ('informing', 'consultation' and 'placation') as degrees of tokenism. Only the top three rungs ('partnership', 'delegated power' and 'citizen control') were classed as degrees of citizen power. *Figure 2.3* shows an adaptation of Arnstein's Ladder, based on Shemmings and Shemmings (1995, p. 52). The latter authors' adaptation illustrates higher and lower degrees of participation and non-participation in community care. Unlike Arnstein, Shemmings and Shemmings consider 'placation' to be a form of non-participation, omit 'therapy' from their ladder, and add 'involvement' as a lower degree of participation.

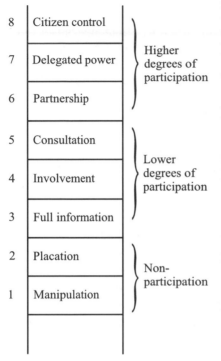

Richardson criticised Arnstein's Ladder and other typologies that differentiate between 'true participation' and 'tokenism' or 'pseudo-participation'. She argued that arrangements for participation do not 'necessarily lead to particular predictable results... The assumption... that the impact of participation will necessarily be of a particular kind is unfounded... The process of bargaining which participation entails makes the result of... dimensions uncertain and unpredictable' (Richardson 1983, p. 93f). In addition, some critiques of tokenism tend to assume that all service users/carers want power and to participate at higher degrees, when research has found that this is not always the case (Byrt 1994, Caress *et al*, 1998). An assumption, for example, that participation limited to information and consultation is always tokenistic, does not

Figure 2.3: Adaptation of Arnstein's Ladder of Participation (1969), based on Shemmings and Shemmings, 1995

consider individual service users' varied views on whether different degrees of participation are empowering or not (see Byrt and Dooher, 2002). For example, for one patient on a surgical ward, the giving of information is disempowering because it does not meet her expectations for participation. For another patient, it increases self-efficacy, and enables him to participate in his care, and perhaps, participate at higher levels and degrees. Barnes and Bowl (2001) argue that some empowerment involves negotiation, partnership or sharing of decisions, rather than shifts in power. They give examples of ways in which individuals can be enabled to make decisions or gain control over their lives, without this necessarily meaning that other people will lose power. Where service users are relatively powerless, individuals may be subversive. Examples include marginalised groups of people, eg. AIDS activists, producing alternative discourses which challenge those of people in positions of power

(Barnes and Bowl, 2001, quoting Altman, 1994, p. 11). Examples of subversion in mental health services include expressing overt agreement with professionals in order to effect discharge, while covertly maintaining an opposed position; and finding ways to bend unreasonable rules to one's advantage, thus 'working the system' (Goffman, 1968; Porter, 1998). In addition, empowerment can be 'reactive', attempting to ameliorate disempowerment within existing services; or 'proactive', with 'service users' setting up and running their own alternative facilities (Barnes and Bowl, 2001). The latter seek to avoid power imbalances and rigid distinctions and barriers between 'providers' and 'users' of services. Examples of such services are given in Chamberlin (1988) and Priestley (1999).

Other typologies of degrees of participation

Brager *et al* (1987) proposed a typology of participation which included 'none [ie. no participation], receives information, advises, plans jointly, has delegated authority and has control' (Tones, 1998a, p. 194, citing Brager and Specht, 1973). *Figure 2.4* illustrates a modification of this typology.

Other earlier typologies of degrees of participation include several related to industry, ranging from workers having little or no influence on decisions to taking complete control (Argyle, 1989; Handy, 1993). Dinkel *et al* (1981) listed, 'seven major categories of activities... representing varying degrees of participation of citizens in community mental health center evaluations'. These included taking part as respondents in surveys, and involvement in planning, conducting and reviewing evaluations and considering programme goals. Participation of service users and carers in different stages of research is considered by Kemshall and Littlechild (2000).

Philpot proposed a 'continuum of user involvement', comprising information, consultation, participation and user control with provision of budgets 'delegated to users to run their own services or carry out pieces of work on behalf of commissioning agencies' (Fraher and Limpinnian, 1999, p. 148, citing Philpot, 1994). Hickey and Kipping's (1998) 'participation continuum' includes information/explanation, consultation, partnership and user control. They argue that:

The first two positions, 'information/explanation' and 'consultation' are more closely associated with the consumerist approach to empowerment, because they do not transfer any decision making to the user. The 'partnership' and 'user control' positions reflect a democratisation approach because power is shifted from the service provider to the service user.

(Hickey and Kipping, 1998, p. 85)

Degree			
High	5	Total running of the organisation	The organisation is run entirely by service users/carers, who decide whether or not to involve other people in decision making
	4	Equal participation	Service users/carers and other participants are equally involved in decision making. There may be little or no distinction between service users/carers and non-service users/carers
	3	Direct representation	One or more service users/carers, representing client/patient/carer opinion, are actively involved in decision making
	2	Consultation	Managers and professionals ask service users/carers their views and opinions and take these into account when making decisions
	1	Information/ explanation	Managers and professionals provide service users/carers with information and explanation of their decisions, but do not otherwise involve them in decision making
Low	0	Nil	All decisions are made entirely by managers and professionals, who do not explain their decisions to service users/carers or involve them in decision making. Clear distinctions between decision makers and service users/carers

Figure 2.4: Degrees of participation (based on Brager *et al*, 1987; Tones, 1998a)

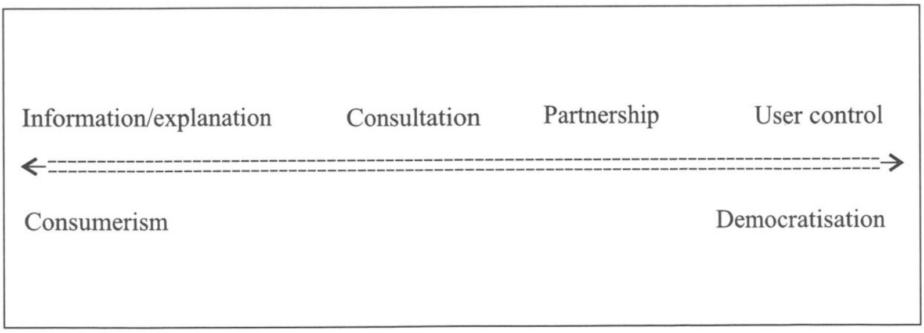

Information/explanation   Consultation   Partnership   User control

←--→

Consumerism   Democratisation

Figure 2.5: Participation continuum of Hickey and Kipping (1998)

Richard Byrt and James Dooher

Various models of professional-service user relationships and decision making have been proposed (Florin and Coulter, 2001; Robinson and Thomson, 2001), including Degner's Scale to assess patients' 'decision making preferences', reflecting degrees of participation in medical consultations (Robinson and Thomson, 2001, p. 36, citing Degner and Sloan, 1992). Degner's scale ranges from decisions made solely by the patient to those where the doctor has total control, and chooses treatment without discussion or consultation with the patient. Byrt and Dooher (2002) consider some of the research on service users'/carers' preferences for degrees of participation.

Levels of participation

The term 'level' is used to refer to the **extent** of individuals' participation or empowerment, ranging from a health service user's involvement in decisions affecting his/her care, to participation in central Government policy making.

Not all typologies of participation include levels. Windle and Cibulka (1981) referred to impacts of participation on political, organisational and service levels. Shields (1985) commented:

> ... participation can be encouraged at various levels. Patients can be involved in choosing and executing a course of treatment; life on psychiatric wards can be influenced by ward community meetings; at a higher level, patients can be consulted and involved in deciding overall policies and plan services...

(Shields, 1985, p. 119)

Figure 2.6 is a proposed typology of levels of participation, based on Byrt (1994). Level 1 concerns the individual: his/her participation and empowerment within a professional-service user/carer relationship, or in the care, services or treatment received. The next level concerns participation affecting a small number of other local health service users/carers. Examples include self-help groups, involvement in decision making or responsibility in voluntary organisations, in a ward, day centre or local community team. Level 3 participation is concerned with participation in part of a trust–wide health service, or part of a social service or voluntary organisation; or involvement, directly or indirectly, in an NHS trust board or its equivalent in the independent sector. Levels 4, 5 and 6 refer to individuals' participation (usually involving actual or attempted influence) at local health authority/local government, regional (eg. regional NHS Executive) and central Government/national levels respectively. These levels also include participation in local, regional and national levels of voluntary organisations. Finally, level 7 refers to participation on a global or 'sub-global' scale, eg. in relation to a continent.

7	**Global** or **'sub-global'**. Individual participates in statutory or voluntary organisations concerned with health issues involving the world as a whole, a continent or other large area of the world (for example, World Health Organization, Health Action International, European Agency for the Evaluation of Medical Products [Hogg, 1999])
6	**National/central Government**. Individual has attempted or actual influence on central Government policy making, eg. through committee or commission membership, or lobbying MPs. In addition or alternatively, participation may be through membership of a national voluntary organisation
5	**Regional**. Individual participates in bodies concerned with a region, eg. regional NHS executive boards, regional social services, inspectorates, membership of regional committees of national voluntary organisation
4	**Local health, social and voluntary services**. Individual participates in local social services committees or in attempts to influence local government councillors or officials. Participation in district health authorities and other bodies at district level, and/or in management of a local voluntary organisations
3	**Large health services/local statutory service subcommittees**. Individual participates in decision making in large health services or at level of NHS trust board or its equivalent in the independent sector; or in social services or voluntary organisation subcommittees
2	**Small groups/health services**. Individual participates in decisions affecting others in a small self-help group, voluntary organisation, small health services, eg. a ward or family practice
1	**Individual**. Individual participates in decisions affecting his/her care, treatment, services or life
0	**No participation/influence at any level**

Figure 2.6: Typology of levels of participation including attempted or actual influence (based on Byrt, 1994)

Mode of intervention

Another dimension of participation is the mode of intervention, a term used by Brager *et al* (1987) to refer to the relationship between service users and decision makers. These authors describe 'collaboration', 'campaigning' and 'contest and disruption'. A distinction has been made between partnership and separatist models of participation, eg. in mental health services run by people with experience as service users (Chamberlin, 1988). In partnership models, service users or carers invite professionals to work with them, while in those which are separatist, professionals or other individuals are refused membership or co-option (Byrt and Lomas, 2001; Chamberlin, 1988). Recent UK mental health survivors' movements have adopted partnership approaches, which contrast with some separatist patients' rights movements in North America. For example, Campbell (1998) described mental health service users' contributions to 'Department of Health reviews and to the House of Commons Select Committee on Health and collaboration with the NHS Executive's Mental Health Task Force' (p. 238).

Oliver and Barnes (1998) distinguished between organisations **of**, and those **for**, people with disabilities. While some of the latter have reinforced stereotypes of disabled people and support the medicalisation of disability, '... the disabled people's movement... [challenges] traditional medical definitions of disability and views that disabled people are incapable, powerless and passive...' (Oliver and Barnes, 1998, p. 71). Organisations **of** disabled people have taken a political stance, sometimes in opposition to central Government policies (Sayce, 2000).

Sanoff (2000) outlines ways to enable consensus building in community participation, but also points out the importance of recognising conflict and developing strategies for its resolution. Tones (1998a) describes two modes of intervention:

> *The first of these consists of more direct and radical social action involving confrontation and protest — and stopping just short of revolution... The second and much more respectable strategy involves the development of community coalitions. It is argued that change is more likely to happen if the coalitions of those who have status, resources and power are formed to combat the substantial influence of government, commercial and other vested interests...*

(Tones 1998a, p. 198, citing Goodman *et al*, 1988)

Smithies and Webster (1998) distinguish between 'top-down' and 'bottom-up' approaches in community participation in health issues. The former have been initiated by central Government and early voluntary organisation efforts to promote self-help; including, for example, some of the work of the Charity Organisation Society in Victorian England (Woodroofe, 1974). Bottom-up approaches to participation have been facilitated by local 'grass roots' organisations which have undertaken political campaigning and mutual aid or self-help activities. In some instances, central or local government and healthcare professionals have worked with these organisations in order to improve health (Roberts, 1998; Smithies and Webster, 1998). Scrambler and Scrambler (1998) refer to the delineation by Rhodes *et al* (1991) of four models 'to inform community-based approaches to health promotion'. Scrambler and Scrambler indicate that 'the information-giving or prevention' and 'self-empowerment' models tend to be top-down, the former being based on professional perspectives, and the self-empowerment model ignoring wider societal influences on health. In contrast, 'community action' and 'radical-political or social transformatory' approaches are bottom-up, with initiatives for action from local individuals and organisations (Scrambler and Scrambler, 1998, p. 120, citing Rhodes *et al*, 1991).

Formal and informal participation

'Formal' participation refers to involvement which is planned, with clear roles and responsibilities (Byrt, 1994). Examples of formal participation include decisions by both nurse and patient that the latter will be involved in all stages of the planning, implementation and evaluation of care. Other examples include designated responsibilities and roles, eg. a service user chairing a community meeting in a mental health unit or serving as a non-executive member of a NHS trust board.

Informal participation refers to unplanned, spontaneous involvement of service users. An example would be a decision made by residents in a nursing home to complain collectively to the matron about conditions, or to hold an impromptu social event and to take on responsibility for its preparation.

Byrt (1994) contrasted formal and informal participation in two voluntary organisations for mental health. In social clubs in one organisation in 'Westhill', participation was informal, unplanned and spontaneous. In one club, in particular, it was difficult to differentiate between 'members' and 'volunteers'; and some respondents saw themselves as occupying both roles, or felt that it was meaningless to distinguish between the two. Participants were keen to avoid making invidious distinctions between participants, or to formalise particular responsibilities. Anyone could decide to perform particular tasks or make decisions, and this was often done in an *ad hoc* way. Attempts by a former participant to impose structure had been firmly rejected.

In contrast, in another voluntary organisation's day centre in 'Eastvale', although some client participation was informal, much of it was formal and characterised by high 'role visibility', ie. it was often clear to a newcomer that a particular day centre member (called a 'steward') was in charge. Stewards had particular, clearly defined responsibilities and tasks, and were responsible for the day centre in the absence of staff. They had a duty rota placed in a prominent position, were the only day centre members allowed access to the kitchen, and were expected to follow certain rules, set and clearly spelt out by the voluntary organisation's officers or the centre manager, to whom they were accountable.

'Conscious' and 'unconscious' participation

Byrt (1994) also distinguished between 'conscious' and 'unconscious' participation. These terms indicate the reasons for, and goals of participation. Conscious participation refers to the involvement of service users in order to facilitate the participation of other individuals with similar health problems or disabilities, and (in some cases) raise their consciousness and/or challenge inadequacies and discrimination in health services and/or wider society (Sayce, 2000). Conscious participation is viewed, at least in part, as an end in itself.

Unconscious participation refers to the involvement of health service users solely or mainly for specific end results, eg. fund raising or the provision of a service. This type of participation does not aim to facilitate the involvement of other health service users, raise their consciousness or challenge services or discrimination (Byrt, 1994).

The voluntary organisation in 'Eastvale' provided an interesting example of a mix of conscious and unconscious participation. The social workers who founded the organisation consciously facilitated the participation of service users from the start because they believed that this would be of benefit. Some members provided opportunities for participation, eg. through open meetings in the organisation's day centre and (in the case of professionals) by deciding to become co-opted, rather than full members of its committee, with a determination not to dominate meetings. On the other hand, much participation was unconscious. For example, a day centre member started a self-help group for people who, like herself, had depression because no such group was available, rather than because she wanted to participate.

Some members who took on responsibility for the day-to-day running of the day centre stressed the extrinsic rewards of their participation, such as payment of a small allowance and access to tea and coffee, rather than the intrinsic benefits of taking on responsibility as a steward for the centre. Within the voluntary organisation, this activity was not described as 'service user participation'. A few respondents in this study indicated that centre users had taken on some responsibilities, not entirely because participants perceived their participation as of value in itself, but to obviate a shortage of 'non-service user' volunteers (Byrt, 1994).

Overt and covert participation

Related to the 'consciousness' or 'unconsciousness' of participation, is the extent to which service users make explicit that this is **because** of their own experience, problem, illness or disability. In overt participation, individuals state that this is the reason for their involvement. They regard their own experience as enabling them to contribute positively to other people in similar situations (Byrt, 1994). This may include campaigning to improve services and in some cases, to reduce oppression and stigmatisation (Barnes and Bowl, 2001; Oliver and Barnes, 1998; Sayce, 2000).

> *If you've experienced paranoia, you know what it's like. If you've seen and heard things which are not there, you know what they're going through.*

> *I was the main instigator [of participation] because of my own experience [of oppression as a mental health patient]... Now I've got allies.*

(Quotes from research interviews in Byrt, 1994)

In contrast, in covert participation, individuals are involved not because of their experience as health service users, but because of other roles or skills that they bring to the organisation.

Overt participation includes 'coming out' for service users who are stigmatised by wider society. In one of the voluntary organisations studied by Byrt (1994), there was a debate about whether members of the national committee should 'come out' and make explicit their former experience as mental health service users. There were mixed views about this issue. Some participants considered that it was a private matter, but others felt that coming out would benefit other service users and make it clear to members of the public that anyone can experience mental health problems. A few years later, several candidates standing for election to this voluntary organisation's national committee made explicit their experience as service users.

The extent to which participation is conscious or unconscious, overt, or covert, depends partly on how service users and carers perceive their roles in health service organisations, and in some cases, in wider society. *Chapter 1* (Byrt and Dooher, 2002), in the companion volume to this book, considers the diverse roles of service users and carers.

The relationship between empowerment and participation

What is the relationship between empowerment and participation? In relation to the four dimensions of empowerment identified on *page 24*, research (including studies referred to in this book) suggests that participation, particularly at higher degrees, is more likely to be successful if the following factors are present:

❖ **Psychological or individual empowerment**. Service users and carers have self-efficacy, including beliefs that they have abilities and skills to participate; and in some circumstances, to effect changes that positively influence their care, the services they receive, or their lives in general. Individuals' expectations about their own roles, and those of professionals, in relation to participation, may also be important, as is their wish to participate (Byrt and Dooher, 2002).

❖ **Service-initiated empowerment**. Professionals and managers are willing, and have the necessary skills (including those related to communication, relationships and leadership) to empower service users and carers, and to enable their participation, eg. in relation to exercising choice or making decisions.

❖ **Empowerment related to service change**. Service users and carers can readily see that their participation results in **actual** changes in care or service provision, whether this is at individual, local or national level.

❖ **Empowerment related to social inclusion and social change**. For many people, particularly service users and carers who are stigmatised in wider society, empowerment and participation within health services may result in little overall personal benefit if they continue to face social exclusion. For some service users and carers, attempts at empowerment and participation will be more meaningful if these endeavour to challenge negative attitudes in wider society; and result in action to ensure a reduction in discrimination, and the same opportunities and choices available to other people.

These, and other factors likely to facilitate and hinder participation and empowerment, are considered by many of the authors in this book and in its companion volume (Dooher and Byrt, 2002a).

Conclusion

This chapter has reviewed definitions and dimensions of empowerment and participation. In the 1960s and 1970s, 'participation' became a 'buzz word', to be replaced in popularity by 'empowerment'.

> *No respectable academic, policy or practitioner discourse is complete without its nod in the direction of the empowered consumer, the empowered citizen or even the empowered worker.*
>
> (Barnes and Warren, 1999, p. 1)

An understanding of the nature and complexity of empowerment and participation can contribute to the successful implementation of strategies to empower service users and carers and enable their participation.

Key points

⌘ Both participation and empowerment have been seen as a 'good thing', but there is a lack of clear definitions and conceptualisation in much of the literature.

⌘ Ideas and strategies for participation and empowerment are often difficult to implement. Implementation may be facilitated by identifying the components, dimensions, degrees and levels of these concepts.

⌘ A model of four dimensions of empowerment is proposed. These include: psychological or individual empowerment; service-initiated empowerment; service change; and social change and social inclusion. Definitions of empowerment in the literature vary in the extent that they include one or more of these dimensions.

⌘ In psychological empowerment, components include increases in self-esteem, self-efficacy and internal locus of control. Psychological empowerment may enable participation and the achievement of change. Components of service-initiated empowerment include aspects of professional-service user/carer relationships and communication; and the extent that professionals are willing to enable or share power.

⌘ The actual achievement of service change empowerment by service users/carers is related to their opportunities for participation; and in a consumerist model, to components of choice, control, autonomy, accessibility, rights and advocacy. In the social change and social inclusion dimension, components include consciousness raising; challenges to oppression, inequality and discrimination; and access to life opportunities.

⌘ A proposed model of participation includes dimensions of degrees and levels of participation; components, types and methods; modes of intervention; types of participant; openness, consciousness and formality.

⌘ Degrees of participation vary from 'none' to 'total control of the organisation.' Several authors have criticised 'tokenism' or 'pseudo-participation', with little or no power devolved to service users or carers. However, research suggests that not all service users and carers want increased power, and some prefer to participate at lower degrees and levels.

⌘ The term 'levels' refers to the extent of individuals' participation or empowerment, ranging from decisions about a client's care to involvement in central Government policy making.

⌘ 'Mode of intervention' describes the relationship between service users/carers and people in positions of power. This may involve collaboration or opposition, separatism or partnership, 'top-down' or 'bottom-up' approaches. A distinction has been made between services 'of' and services 'for' clients.

⌘ Participation can be formal, with clear roles and responsibilities, or informal and spontaneous. It can be conscious, with participation as an end in itself, but often with goals of consciousness raising or challenging services or social perceptions. In contrast, unconscious participation does not have these aims. Participants are not primarily involved because of their service user/carer experience; and their participation is concerned mainly with concrete end results, such as fund raising and service provision.

⌘ Participation can also be overt, with individuals making it clear that their participation is based on their experience as a service user or carer, often in order to contribute to others in similar situations. Overt participation may involve 'coming out' and challenging stigmatisation. In covert participation, individuals do not make explicit their 'service user' or 'carer' experiences.

References

Argyle M (1989) *The Social Psychology of Work*. 2nd edn. Penguin Books, Harmondsworth

Arnstein S (1969) A Ladder of Citizen Participation. *Am Institute of Planners J* **3**(Part 4): 216

Barnes M, Bowl R (2001) *Taking Over the Asylum. Empowerment and Mental Health*. Palgrave, Basingstoke

Barnes M, Warren L (1999) Introduction. In: Barnes M, Warren L, eds. (1999) *Paths to Empowerment*. The Policy Press, University of Bristol, Bristol

Boaden N, Goldsmith M, Hampton W, Stringer P (1982) *Public Participation in Local Services*. Longman, London

Bracht N, Kingsbury L, Rissel C (1999) A five-stage community organisation model for health promotion. In: Bracht N, ed. (1999) *Health Promotion at the Community Level 2. New Advances*. Sage Publications, Thousand Oaks, CA: chap 4

Brager G, Specht H, Torczyner JL (1987) *Community Organising*. 2nd edn. Columbia University Press, New York

Braye S (2000) Participation and Involvement in Social Care: An Overview. In: Kemshall and Littlechild (2000), *op cit*: chap 1

Braye S, Preston-Shoot M (1995) *Empowering Practice in Social Care.* Open University Press, Buckingham

Byrt R (1994) *Consumer Participation in a Voluntary Organisation for Mental Health.* Unpublished PhD Thesis, Loughborough University, Loughborough

Byrt R (2001) Power, influence and control in practice development. In: Clark A, Dooher J, Fowler J, eds. (2001). *Handbook of Practice Development.* Quay Books, Mark Allen Publishing Limited, Dinton, Salisbury: chap 10

Byrt R, Dooher J (2002) Service users and their desire for empowerment and participation. In: Dooher J, Byrt R (2002), *op cit:* chap 1

Byrt R, Lomas C (2001) Women's Secure Services in the UK. In: Landsberg G, Smiley A, eds. *Forensic Mental Health. Working with Offenders with Mental Illness.* Civic Research Institute, Kingston, NJ: chap 38

Cahill J (1998) Patient participation – A review of the literature. *J Clin Nurs* **7**: 119–28

Campbell P (1998) Listening to clients. In: Barker P, Davidson B, eds. (1998) *Psychiatric Nursing. Ethical Strife.* Arnold, London: chap 17

Caress AL *et al* (1998) Patient-sensitive treatment decision making? Preferences and perceptions of a sample of renal patients. *NT Research* **3**(5): 364–72

Chamberlin J (1988) *On Our Own. Patient Controlled Alternatives to the Mental Health System.* MIND Publications, London

Chamberlin J (1997) A working definition of empowerment. *Psychiatric Rehabilitation J* **20**(4): 43–6

Cormack DFS, ed. (2000) *The Research Process in Nursing.* 4th edn. Blackwell Science, Oxford

Coulter A (1997) Partnerships with patients: the pros and cons of shared clinical decision-making. *J Health Serv Res* **2**: 112–21

Coulter A, Entwhistle V, Gilbert D (1998) *Informing Patients.* King's Fund, London

Dinkel NR, Zinober JW, Flaherty EW (1981) Citizen participation in CMHC programme evaluation. A neglected potential. *Community Ment Health J* **17**(Part 1): 54–7

Department of Health (1992) *The Health of the Nation: A Strategy for Health in England.* HMSO, London, Cmnd 1986

Department of Health (1998a) *A First Class Service: Quality in the New NHS.* DoH, London

Department of Health (1998b) *Saving Lives. Our Healthier Nation.* DoH, London

Dooher J, Byrt R (2002a) *Empowerment and the the Health Service User.* Quay Books, Mark Allen Publishing Limited, Dinton, Salisbury: chap 1

Dooher J, Byrt R (2002b) Conclusions. In: Dooher J, Byrt R (2002a) *op cit*

Draper P (1997) *Nursing Perspectives on Quality of Life.* Routledge, London

Fatchett A (1998) *Nursing in the New NHS, Modern, Dependable?* Baillière Tindall, London

Faulkner M (2001) A measure of patient empowerment in hospital environments catering for older people. *J Adv Nurs* **34**(5): 676–86

Florin D, Coulter A (2001) Partnership in the primary care consultation. In: Gillam S, Brooks F, eds. (2001) *New Beginnings. Towards Patient and Public Involvement in Primary Health Care.* King's Fund/University of Luton, London: chap 4

Fraher A, Limpinnian M (1999) User Empowerment Within Mental Health Nursing. In: Wilkinson G, Miers M (1999) *op cit:* chap 10

Gale J (1998) Learning disability: dimension of professional empowerment. *J Learning Disability Health and Social Care* **2**(2): 110–15

Gibson CH (1995) The process of empowerment in mothers of chronically disabled children. *J Adv Nurs* **21**: 1201–10

Gillibrand W, Flynn M (2001) Forced externalisation of control in people with diabetes: a qualitative exploratory study. *J Adv Nurs* **34**(4): 501–10

Godfrey J (2002) Empowerment and participation. The lesbian, gay man's and transgendered experience as users of healthcare services. In: Dooher J, Byrt R (2002) *op cit:* chap 6

Goffman E (1968) *Asylums. Essays on the Social Situation of Mental Patients and Others.* Penguin Books, Harmondsworth

Green J, Tones K (2002) The creative arts and empowerment. In: Dooher J, Byrt R (2002) *op cit*

Handy CB (1993) *Understanding Organisations.* 2nd edn. Penguin Books, Harmondsworth

Hickey G, Kipping C (1998) Exploring the concepts of user involvements in mental health through a participation continuum. *J Psychiatric Ment Health Nurs* **7**: 83–8

Hogg C (1999) *Patients, Power and Politics. From Patients to Citizens.* Sage Publications, London

Jackson A (1997) *Oppression and Empowerment. The Scope for Praxis in Mental Health.* MA dissertation. De Montfort University, Leicester

Jackson A, Hislop J (2002) User empowerment and involvement in mental health. In: Dooher J, Byrt, R (2002) *op cit*: chap 2

Kemshall H, Littlechild R, eds. (2000) *User Involvement and Participation in Social Care. Research Informing Practice.* Jessica Kingsley, London

Kendall S, ed. (1998a) *Health and Empowerment. Research and Practice.* Arnold, London

Kendall S (1998b) Introduction. In: Kendall S, ed. (1998a) *op cit*

Kennedy LA (2001) Community involvement at what cost? Local appraisal of a pan-European nutrition promotion programme in low-income neighbourhoods. *Health Promotion International* **16**(1): 35–44

Kuokkanen L, Leino-Kilpi H (2000) Power and empowerment in nursing: three theoretical approaches. *J Adv Nurs* **31**(1): 235–41

Laverack G, Wallerstein N (2001) Measuring Community empowerment: a fresh look at organizational domains. *Health Promot Internation* **16**(2): 179–85

Leskell JK, Johansson I, Wibell LB, Wikblad KF (2001) Power and self-perceived health in blind diabetic and non-diabetic individuals. *J Adv Nurs* **34**(4): 511–20

Lupton C, Peckham S, Taylor P (1998) *Managing Public Involvement in Healthcare Purchasing.* Open University Press, Buckingham

Mason T, Carlisle C, Watkins C, Whitehead E, eds (2001) *Stigma and Social Exclusion in Healthcare.* Routledge, London

McFadyen J, Farrington A (1997) User and carer participation in the NHS. *Br J Health Care Management* **3**(5): 260–4

Melluish S (1998) Community psychology. A social action approach to psychological distress. In: Barker P, Davidson B, eds. *Psychiatric Nursing. Ethical Strife.* Arnold, London: chap 19

Midgley J, Hall A, Hardiman M, Narine N (1986) *Community Participation, Social Development and the State.* Methuen, London

Miers M (1999) Health teams in the community. In: Wilkinson G, Miers M (1999) *op cit*: chap 8

Oliver M, Barnes M (1998) *Disabled People and Social Policy: From Exclusion to Inclusion.* Longman, London

Paterson B (2001) Myth of Empowerment in Chronic Illness. *J Adv Nurs* **34**(5): 574–81

Porter S (1998) The social interpretation of deviance. In: Birchenall M, Birchenall P, eds. *Sociology as Applied to Nursing and Health Care.* Baillière Tindall in association with the Royal College of Nursing, London: chap 7

Priestley M (1999) *Disability Politics and Community Care.* Jessica Kingsley, London

Richardson A (1983) *Participation.* Routledge and Kegan Paul, London

Roberts H (1998) Empowering communities. The case of childhood accidents. In: Kendall S, ed. *Health and Empowerment. Research and Practice.* Arnold, London: chap 6

Robinson A, Thomson R (2001) Variability in patient preferences for participating in medical decision making: implication for the use of decision support tools. *Qual Health Care* **10**(suppl I): 34–8

Rodwell CM (1996) An analysis of the concept of empowerment. *J Adv Nurs* **23**(2): 305–13

Sanoff H (2000) *Community Participation. Methods in Design and Planning.* John Wiley, New York

Sayce L (2000) *From Psychiatric Patient to Citizen. Overcoming Discrimination and Social Exclusion.* Macmillan, Basingstoke

Scrambler G, Scrambler A (1998) Women sex workers, health promotion and HIV. In: Kendall S (1998a) *op cit*: chap 5

Shaw I (2000) Just inquiry? Research and evaluation for service users. In: Kemshall H, Littlechild R (2000) *op cit*: chap 2

Shemmings, D, Shemmings Y(1995) Defining participative practice in health and welfare.In: Jack R, ed. *Empowerment in Community Care.* Chapman and Hall, London: chap 2

Shields PJ (1985) The consumer's view of psychiatry. *Hosp Health Serv Rev* **81**(3): 117–9

Shiffman J (2002) The construction of community participation: village family planning groups and the Indonesian state. *Soc Sci Med* **54**: 1199–1214

Skelton R (1994) Nursing and empowerment: concepts and strategies. *J Adv Nurs* **19**: 415–23

Smithies J, Webster G (1998) *Community Involvement in Health. From Passive Recipients to Active Participants.* Ashgate, Aldershot

Teasdale K (1998) *Advocacy in Health Care.* Blackwell Science, Oxford

Richard Byrt and James Dooher

Tones K (1998a) Empowerment for health: the challenge. In: Kendall S, ed. *Health and Empowerment, Research and Practice*. Arnold, London: chap 9

Tones K (1998b) Health education and the promotion of health: seeking wisely to empower. In: Kendall S (1998a) *op cit*: chap 3

Wilkinson G (1999) Theories of power. In: Wilkinson G, Miers M (1999) *op cit*: chap 1

Wilkinson G, Miers M, eds (1999) *Power and Nursing Practice*. Macmillan, Basingstoke

Windle C, Cibulka J (1981) A framework for understanding participation in community mental health services. *Community Ment Health J* **17** (part 1)

Woodroofe K (1974) *From Charity to Social Work in England and the United States*. Routledge and Kegan Paul, London

3

Empowerment, participation and the rise of orthodox biomedicine

Mike Saks

Introduction

This chapter aims to shed light on public participation and empowerment by examining developments in health care from the sixteenth century onwards, primarily focusing on Britain. It covers pre-industrial medicine, the rise of orthodox biomedicine, the changes that have taken place in health care in the contemporary context and the challenges that lay ahead in this field. Although these areas are dealt with chronologically in general terms, the main theme of the chapter is that the growth of orthodox biomedicine, for all its associated health benefits, has posed a major challenge to the participation and empowerment of the consumer. Indeed, it is argued that this challenge continues to exist despite the many recent reforms in health care in this country that have helped to re-shape its boundaries. The chapter is based on a keynote address made at a conference on 'Healthcare for the Whole Person' held at the Royal Society of Medicine in London on 11–12 October, 2000.

The notion of participation and empowerment has been conceived in many ways, but in this context is essentially seen as being that of active engagement enabling people to take control of their own health (Kendall, 1998). To understand the extent of the challenge presented by the development of biomedicine, it is important to recognise that there are a number of models of health care. Even orthodox biomedicine is not set in tablets of stone, as the form that it takes is subject to change over time. The diversity of approaches in relation to participation and empowerment is particularly accentuated when the reductionism inherent in the biomedical approach is contrasted with more holistic systems of health care. These involve the whole person in promoting health and preventing illness, including mind and body, as well as the socio-cultural milieux in which people are located (see, for instance, Gordon, 1996).

Historical background: the empowering holistic tradition

The development of medicine in Britain from the sixteenth to the mid-nineteenth century is initially traced in this chapter. In so doing, it highlights the more holistic forms of medicine practised in this period — which were increasingly transcended as orthodox bio-medicine began to emerge. In this respect, sixteenth century health care was extremely diverse, including, among other things, the use of charms, incantations, plants and minerals. In terms of empowerment, most of this was based on local self-help, in which stress was placed on self-responsibility for health. Self-help was normally practised out of neighbourliness and religious duty, and was aimed at ensuring a balanced constitution in terms of diet and exercise (Porter, 1995). If this indicates the early importance given to public participation in health, it should also be emphasised that there was a growing array of practitioners involved in health care (Larner, 1992).

These included a wide range of exponents of health care, from herbalists to healers. They had different levels of training, reward and commitment and were drawn from both males and females, ministering to a diverse clientele. They encompassed a small number of upper class physicians serving the aristocracy, who gained a monopoly of practice in London from 1518 onwards; the barber-surgeons who were engaged in craft skills such as tooth extraction, manipulation and amputation; and the more lowly apothecaries who separated from the grocers in the seventeenth century and increasingly became independent practitioners rather than simply dispensing for the physicians. It should be remembered that the physicians, surgeons and apothecaries were minority practitioners at this time, whose training was heavily based on the apprenticeship model. They had yet to move to the centre of the healthcare stage, even if they gained ever greater authority as time progressed in the healthcare division of labour (Stevens, 1966).

Although such practitioners might be seen as reducing public involvement in their own care — especially since a large measure of secrecy was involved in giving treatment — much health activity in this period was underpinned by empowering holistic philosophies. This is illustrated by the mind-body links involved in common practices like the laying on of hands, the reciting of words and the wearing of amulets to ward off suffering (Larner, 1992). Even the frequently employed practices of purging, sweating, vomiting and bloodletting aimed at restoring bodily equilibrium, based on the medieval notion of balancing the humours, often involved the consumer. This was especially accentuated in relation to physicians consulting with rich higher status clients, where the diagnosis and type of intervention used was heavily influenced by the wishes of individual fee-paying patients in the patronage system of 'bedside medicine' that had emerged by the eighteenth century (Jewson, 1974).

It is important not to idealise this period in terms of client participation and control. The health practices employed were not necessarily the most effective in controlling illness and disease — whatever the role played by the consumer. This is illustrated by their lack of success in warding off the contemporary scourge of the plague (Larner, 1992). Nor were they always very safe, as highlighted by some of the debilitating effects of the heroic therapies that were used (Porter, 1995). There were also undoubtedly some practitioners who defrauded their clientele in publicising spurious nostrums for pecuniary gain and prescribed remedies empirically without regard to their rationale (Maple, 1992). Nonetheless, the holistic thrust of much of the pluralistic system of health care of the day is clear — even if the boundaries between orthodoxy and unorthodoxy were still relatively indistinct (Saks, 1992). The important role played by the public is underlined by the way in which client demand was reflected in the competitive marketplace for the ever broader range of therapies that emerged in the eighteenth century, as capitalism developed (Porter, 1989).

The empowering holistic aspects of this healthcare system were increasingly left behind with the rise of modern biomedicine. This was centred on the philosophical mind-body split attributed to Descartes, in which the body was viewed like a machine, separate from the mind whose parts were viewed as needing to be repaired on malfunction (Saks, 1997a). The first phase of this process involved physicians, surgeons and apothecaries moving from local to legally recognised national bodies as the eighteenth century wore on (Stevens, 1966). Greater unity then developed between the three branches of medicine in the first half of the nineteenth century as they sought professional standing based on exclusionary social closure. One consequence of this was the increase in standardisation of medical education around practice-focused biomedical competence, linked to the establishment of hospital medical schools and growing advances in fields like surgery (Cule, 1997).

The rise of orthodox biomedicine: the disempowered consumer

A crucial landmark in this process was the 1858 Medical Registration Act, which formalised the unification of medicine, laid down minimum educational standards, underwrote the concept of professional self-regulation, established disciplinary procedures within the new profession and provided protection of title for medical doctors (Saks, 1998). This Act signalled the rise of biomedicine, primarily based on interventions using drugs and surgery, in which the body came to be seen as a symptom-bearing organism. This development was predicated on the emergence of 'hospital medicine', which increasingly replaced the more holistic framework of 'bedside medicine'. This was marked by growing medical interest in classifying disease generically, as opposed to dealing holistically with individual cases. The next step was the growth of 'laboratory medicine' in which the body was progressively conceived as being made up of a complex of cells (Jewson, 1976).

The consequence of this from the viewpoint of participation and empowerment was that the newly conceived 'patient' was further alienated from the medical profession, whose membership to compound matters was predominantly male (Witz, 1992). This was because the subjective opinions of the consumer became of even less relevance and diagnosis was increasingly based on the analysis of body samples by technicians who were far removed from personal contact with the patient, and often even geographically at some distance (Jewson, 1976). This objectification of the patient came to form a cornerstone of the paradigm of 'scientific' medicine that was embedded in medical practice and research by the first half of the twentieth century. The rise of biomedicine in these terms was also reinforced at this time by the development of the orthodox healthcare division of labour to include such subordinated groups as nurses, midwives, pharmacists and, a little later, the professions supplementary to medicine (Saks, 1998).

The other significant aspect of the development of modern orthodox 'scientific' medicine as far as the demise of more holistic practice was concerned was the successful attack launched by leaders of the medical profession between the early nineteenth century and the mid-twentieth century on groups that had increasingly become re-defined as alternative practitioners. These included groups like the hydropaths and homeopaths who often subscribed to holistic philosophies about mind, body and the stimulation of the life force in practices based on the active engagement and participation of the consumer. The attack on such practitioners ranged from negative diatribes against 'quackery' in the medical journals to sanctions against deviants within the profession itself. This seems to have reduced the numbers of alternative practitioners and limited to some degree the use of unorthodox therapies in the self-help context (Saks, 1996).

While this attack was undertaken under the banner of scientific progress, it could be seen — like the process of professionalisation itself — as a political attempt by the developing medical elite to strengthen its power, status and income by limiting competition from occupational rivals allowed to practise under the Common Law. This seems to be a more plausible explanation of the assault on the medical alternatives than one based on a profession dedicated to advancing the public interest at this stage. In the latter half of the nineteenth century doctors were still using heroic therapies. Antiseptic and aseptic techniques had not yet been fully implemented and hospitals were seen as 'gateways to death' by the working class (Saks, 1994). This can scarcely be viewed, therefore, as a framework that was strongly engaging and empowering consumers in the health arena — even if medical advice was not always taken by members of the public and a few doctors themselves were converts to alternative therapies (see, for example, Nicholls, 1988).

Having said this, in terms of controlling health, it would be wrong to deny the benefits that have subsequently derived from more developed forms of biomedicine. These include such innovations as the discovery of insulin for diabetics, the use of antibiotics, blood transfusions, hip replacements and cataract surgery (Duin and Sutcliffe, 1992). These treatments have saved lives and improved the quality of life for large numbers of people, especially as growing state support has enhanced access to services in the twentieth century through such mechanisms as the 1911 National Health Insurance Act and the 1946 National Health Service Act in Britain (Allsop, 1995). It is argued though, that while modern biomedicine has contributed to human health, its achievements are more limited than often supposed.

This was very apparent in the late 1960s and 1970s when the notion of scientific progress came under serious challenge in the wake of the growth of a counter culture, aimed in part at enhancing participation and empowerment. This highlighted, among other things, the counterproductive effects of modern medicine (as set out by Illich, 1977). It particularly led to attacks on high technology medicine for dehumanising the patient, giving rise to iatrogenic illnesses and being less effective than its proponents claimed. Classic examples cited by critics included the alienation of those receiving kidney dialysis, the destructive side-effects of thalidomide in pregnant women, and the restricted value of radical mastectomies for breast cancer, given evidence on outcomes and the stigmatisation involved (see, for example, Saks, 2000).

This attack on the limitations of modern medicine, based on the development of alternative lifestyles, went beyond simply challenging the role of the professional expert in health. It was amplified by an increasing awareness of the importance of the wider socio-political environment. In this respect, the impact on health of factors outside medicine such as adequate diet, housing and sanitation were brought into focus (see, for instance, McKeown, 1979). Wider political influences on health were also underlined, not least by the release of the Black Report in Britain in the early 1980s that showed a relationship between class inequalities and health (Townsend *et al*, 1992). These were reinforced by claims about the negative influence of industrial and financial capital on health, including that of the multinational pharmaceutical companies (Doyal, 1979). This led to the questioning of how much, if any, scientific progress had really taken place in modern medicine and even the meaning of the concept of 'science' itself.

Underlying much of this critique was the lack of engagement and empowerment of the consumer. Related issues were also raised in the 1970s and 1980s about whether the predominant biomedical focus on the body, as distinct from the mind-body interface, was improving human health. At this time, public demand for complementary and alternative medicine was taking off, both in terms of self-help and the use of unorthodox practitioners, not least because of growing contact between countries in the East and West (Saks, 1997b). The response of leaders of the medical profession, remained defensive, resulting in an escalating attack on more holistic complementary and alternative therapists. This led to the denigration of the work of practitioners like acupuncturists and aromatherapists, with career obstacles often being placed in the path of sympathisers within the medical profession itself (Saks, 1996). Indeed, the report of the British Medical Association (1986) on alternative therapy spent almost as much time charting the successful march of scientific medical progress, as in condemning most of the alternatives for basing their practice on witchcraft and the supernatural.

Moving forward: contemporary changes in health care in Britain

This stance may have been partly explicable in terms of the perceived risk to the public, in view of the relative lack of training of many of those involved in delivering complementary and alternative medicine at this stage (Fulder, 1996). However, the language used by the medical establishment was inflammatory and did not adequately reflect either areas in which the work of complementary and alternative therapists was more strongly founded or, indeed, biomedicine's own failings. These are especially apparent in dealing with chronic conditions that are often seen as one of the strengths of unorthodox medicine (Saks, 1994). This led some critics to view the defensiveness of mainstream medical bodies largely as a manifestation of their self-interest, in light of the challenge posed to their privileges by rivals outside the ranks of medical orthodoxy. This challenge was augmented by the fact that complementary and alternative practitioners without orthodox qualifications could still practice without the restrictions in place in much of continental Europe (Huggon and Trench, 1992).

Significantly, the past few years in Britain have been marked by change, with the re-emergence of an empowering approach to health care in which people are more fully engaged. This has been, in part, as a result of pressure from consumers, including the women's movement and patient activist groups, as well as political lobbies. These have variously led to the further development of Community Health Councils, the increased lay membership of the General Medical Council and the Patients' Charter (Saks, 2000). From the viewpoint of current Government policy, the public lies at the heart of health care. In this sense, official support is at present being given for everything from a new patient advocacy service in every NHS Trust and the development of patients' forums and citizens' panels, to the more central involvement of the user in research and development in the NHS (Department of Health [DoH], 2000). This clearly represents a sea change from previous policy on consumer engagement.

Moreover, lobbies such as the All-Party Parliamentary Group for Alternative and Complementary Medicine have not allowed the Government to relax in terms of alternative therapies (Saks, 1992). It has also become hard to ignore Prince Charles and other prominent figures who have taken up the cause of integrated medicine, and even more difficult to avoid the voices of the many members of the public who now use its various forms (Sharma, 1995). These, and other trends, have helped to take biomedicine in a more holistic direction based on a more person-centred, inter-professional approach to health care, with greater stress on self-care and patient-practitioner reciprocity (Pietroni, 1991). Given the growing emphasis that has been placed on the wider environment in which the client is located, Western medicine can no longer be stereotyped as being mechanistic and reductionist, as some of its critics would have us believe.

The more holistic development of modern biomedicine is well exemplified by shifts in relation to complementary and alternative medicine. This was signalled in a follow-up report brought out by the British Medical Association (1993) which, far from condemning the growing ranks of outsiders, urged greater collaboration with non-conventional practitioners, especially in non-invasive areas of practice with randomised controlled trial evidence. In addition to the spiralling numbers of nurses, physiotherapists and others turning to this field, close to one in five general practitioners themselves today use complementary and alternative medicine and two in five general practices offer access to such therapies. Most pain clinics and hospices also now employ acupuncture as a matter of routine, with the deployment of aromatherapy and massage rapidly spreading in the acute sector (Burne, 2000). This trend is likely to continue as many types of complementary and alternative medicine professionalise, not least by extending their educational base. This helps to make their work more legitimate, as highlighted by osteopaths and chiropractors who both won the legal right to title, based on the establishment of a statutory register, in the 1990s (Saks, 1999).

In terms of patient empowerment, greater stress is currently being placed on collaborative inter-professional working for the benefit of the consumer in orthodox forms of health care in Britain. This initially developed through the expansion of a hierarchical division of labour, including nurses and other health professions subordinated to medicine. This has now moved forward under the impetus of Government policy to include more equal partnership working between doctors and other health personnel in primary care groups (PCGs) and NHS trusts. The ensuing shift in relationships is symbolised in the projected change of name of the Council for the Professions Supplementary to Medicine to the new Health Professions Council (JM Consulting, 1996). Such changes, as a result of the Government's commitment to encourage more 'joined up' thinking

(DoH, 1997), have begun to encompass more extensive working with the social care area.

There are also flagship areas for partnership working with complementary and alternative therapists, as exemplified by the Bristol Cancer Help Centre and the Marylebone Centre (Pietroni, 1991). These examples help to demonstrate that the moves towards more participative and empowering holistic approaches to health care are increasingly being embraced by Western medicine in terms of inter-professional collaboration. They complement recent efforts to enhance the communication skills of doctors and other orthodox healthcare practitioners in dealing with patients (Saks, 1997a). More whole-person medicine has also been developed through the growing recognition by such personnel of the importance of the social networks in which their clients are embedded, spawning greater involvement by welfare professionals like social workers and counsellors (Leathard, 1994). This is paralleled by the development of public health policy over the last decade that has, among other things; fostered health promotion, made more self-conscious links between health and the environment, and given greater emphasis to combatting wider patterns of social exclusion in health (Baggott, 2000).

Challenges for the future: towards greater participation and empowerment in health care

What challenges for the future lie ahead in relation to empowerment and public participation in health care? One key challenge is to guard against complacency. Much has been achieved in resurrecting some of the threads of the holistic approaches that were evident in Britain two or three centuries ago — before orthodox biomedicine gained ascendance from the nineteenth century onwards — and extending these further. However, it also needs to be recognised that much remains to be done. Modern medicine is still far from providing health care holistically for fully empowered and participating clients. This is evident in areas such as inter-professional working and public health where theory in many cases remains significantly distant from practice despite recent Government initiatives (as illustrated by Leathard, 1994; Baggott, 2000).

A useful barometer of the distance still to be travelled is that of complementary and alternative medicine. Although positive changes have occurred, such therapies remain marginalised in terms of mainstream education and research in health care in this country, especially in their more holistic forms (Saks, 1992). Moreover, the medical incorporation of such therapies is less extensive than first meets the eye. This process often occurs too selectively in terms of both the practices concerned and the scope of their employment. For example, acupuncture has tended to be employed by doctors in Britain in recent times as an analgesic, based on Western-style theories about the release of endorphins (Saks, 1995). This approach means that wider areas of application centred on Oriental yin-yang philosophies may not be adequately explored. Most significantly in this case, it abstracts this form of complementary and alternative therapy from the holistic context of traditional chinese medicine. This may be a loss in so far as the latter encourages non-hierarchical relationships between patients and practitioners, based on the active involvement of patients in their treatment; in which the expert aids the interpretation of their experiences without negating their subjectivity (Busby, 1996).

The reasons for the above situation are complex, but are not unrelated to the interests of leading figures in biomedical orthodoxy in maintaining and enhancing their power, status and income. In this sense, the current medical policy of incorporating rather than condemning complementary and alternative therapies may not so much represent an opening up of boundaries, as an interest-based strategy to inhibit an increasingly serious threat from outsiders with a competing knowledge base. This strategy carries the bonus for orthodox practitioners of facilitating the limited colonisation of selected areas under the banner of biomedicine, which enables them to capitalise on their popularity among the public, while minimising the risks to their own position (Saks, 1995). The cost to the public is that the original holistic philosophies may be lost. This raises critical questions about how far participation and empowerment can be cultivated as long as biomedicine remains in the ascendance.

It should also be noted that, while the number of complementary and alternative therapists in this country outstrips that of general practitioners (Mills and Budd, 2000), holism is not always fully translated into practice even by those operating outside of the orthodox health professions. This applies at a number of levels, including the frequently limited existence of internal and external colleague referral networks; the increasingly biomedical under-pinnings of unorthodox practice; and the relative rarity with which wider factors like poor housing and unemployment are taken into account in addressing the situation of clients (Saks, 1997a). The explanation of this is not disassociated from the hegemonic position of biomedicine and the interests that sustain it. This is because the stake that many complementary and alternative therapists have in gaining legitimacy may make them more cautious about subscribing to holistic models of mind-body medicine. This is particularly crucial at a time when the medical establishment is stressing the need for greater medical control, and a stronger biomedical base for complementary and alternative therapies (British Medical Association, 1993) as practitioners of such therapies seek state sanction in their increasing efforts to professionalise (Saks, 1999).

Interests related to power, income and status may also deleteriously affect other critical areas related to participation and empowerment in orthodox health care. Their influence extends to the medicalisation of self-help (Vincent, 1992) and restrictions on the amount and form of inter-professional collaboration, in which professional tribalism frequently comes into play (Beattie, 1995). Commercial interests also continue heavily to shape the public health agenda to our detriment (Baggott, 2000). To recognise such interests within medicine in Britain is at the heart of the task of developing levers to bring about a more integrated health system, which the public can own more fully and be engaged in creating. If the public are to be the overall beneficiaries, this will involve balancing the advantages of biomedicine — with its exciting modern diagnostic and therapeutic technologies in areas spanning from genetics to micro-surgery — against the straitjacket imposed by its own limitations.

Herein lies the greatest challenge for the future, as there remains a fundamental tension between the emphasis on specialisation and the objectification of the client implicit in biomedicine, and the potential liberation from such conceptions provided by more holistic frames of reference. The rise of biomedical orthodoxy, which has led clients to be treated simply as patients with a generic illness or disease, has undoubtedly diminished the influence of consumers. They have tended to be reduced to a position of dependency, rather than being given more control in relation to their own health care. As has been seen, this has only been modified to some degree by recent healthcare reforms. The opportunity now more than ever exists to draw more fully on the holistic philosophical roots that form part of the historical context of Western medicine. It is vital that this opportunity is not lost if a system of integrated health care, with more public participation and empowerment, is to emerge in this country.

Key points

- ⌘ Significant parallels may be drawn between sixteenth century values and aspirations for health care today. This suggests that our ambitions and ideals have remained stagnant over time and we have progressed little in terms of reaching health goals.

- ⌘ The swift but faltering progress of science and technology has resulted in a raft of mistakes. These mistakes add fuel to the political and cultural demand for safety in the practice of health care, and a more demanding public will consequently hold more power.

- ⌘ Empowerment and participation is a fundamental prerequisite within holistic care, yet biomedicine appears to view both empowerment and participation as an addendum, helpful, but not essential.

- ⌘ A sea change for the health consumer has been driven by a desire for safety, and the emergence of public accountability for health professionals. Orthodox biomedicine has adopted a competitive and largely intolerant stance towards holism, which wastes resources and stifles growth.

- ⌘ Challenges for the future must include an acceptance from traditionalists that alternative and complementary interventions have an equal role to play in creating a truly balanced healthcare system.

References

Allsop J (1995) *Health Policy and the NHS: Towards 2000*. 2nd edn. Longman, London

Baggott R (2000) *Public Health: Policy and Politics*. Macmillan, Basingstoke

Beattie A (1995) War and peace among the health tribes. In: Soothill K, Mackay L, Webb C, eds. *Interprofessional Relations in Health Care*. Edward Arnold, London

British Medical Association (1986) *Report of the Board of Science and Education on Alternative Therapy*. BMA, London

British Medical Association (1993) *Complementary Medicine: New Approaches to Good Practice*. BMA, London

Burne J (2000) Healing in harmony. *The Guardian*, 26 February

Busby H (1996) Alternative medicines/alternative knowledge: Putting flesh on the bones (using traditional Chinese approaches to healing). In: Cant S, Sharma U, eds. *Complementary and Alternative Medicines: Knowledge in Practice*. Free Association Books, London

Cule J (1997) The history of medicine. In: Porter R, ed. *Medicine: A History of Healing*. Ivy Press, London

Department of Health (1997) *The new NHS — modern, dependable*. DoH, London

Department of Health (2000) *The NHS Plan*. DoH, London

Doyal L (1979) *Political Economy of Health*. Pluto Press, London

Duin N, Sutcliffe J (1992) *A History of Medicine: From Pre-history to the Year 2020.* Simon and Schuster, London

Fulder S (1996) *The Handbook of Alternative and Complementary Medicine.* 3rd edn. Oxford University Press, Oxford

Gordon J (1996) *Manifesto for a New Medicine.* Perseus Books, Reading

Huggon T, Trench A (1992) Brussels post-1992: Protector or persecutor? In: Saks M, ed. *Alternative Medicine in Britain.* Clarendon Press, Oxford

Illich I (1977) *Limits to Medicine.* Penguin Books, Harmondsworth

Jewson N (1974) Medical knowledge and the patronage system in eighteenth century England. *Sociology* **8**: 369–85

Jewson N (1976) The disappearance of the sick-man from medical cosmology 1770–1870. *Sociology* **10**: 225–44

JM Consulting (1996) *The Regulation of Health Professions: Report of a Review of the Professions Supplementary to Medicine Act (1960) with Recommendations for New Legislation.* JM Consulting Ltd, Bristol

Kendall S (1998) Introduction. In: Kendall S, ed. *Health and Empowerment: Research and Practice.* Arnold, London

Larner C (1992) Healing in pre-industrial Britain. In: Saks M, ed. *Alternative Medicine in Britain.* Clarendon Press, Oxford

Leathard A, ed. (1994) *Going Inter-professional: Working Together for Health and Welfare.* Routledge, London

McKeown T (1979) *The Role of Medicine: Dream, Mirage or Nemesis?* Basil Blackwell, Oxford

Maple E (1992) The great age of quackery. In: Saks M, ed. *Alternative Medicine in Britain.* Oxford University Press, Oxford

Mills S, Budd S (2000) *Professional Organisation of Complementary and Alternative Medicine in the United Kingdom: A Second Report to the Department of Health.* University of Exeter, Exeter

Nicholls P (1988) *Homeopathy and the Medical Profession.* Croom Helm, London

Pietroni P (1991) *The Greening of Medicine.* Victor Gollancz, London

Porter R (1989) *Health for Sale: Quackery in England 1660–1850.* Manchester University Press, Manchester

Porter R (1995) *Disease, Medicine and Society, 1550–1860.* 2nd edn. Cambridge University Press, Cambridge

Saks M (1992) Introduction. In: Saks M, ed. *Alternative Medicine in Britain.* Oxford University Press, Oxford

Saks M (1994) The alternatives to medicine. In: Gabe J, Kelleher D, Williams G, eds. *Challenging Medicine.* Routledge, London

Saks M (1995) *Professions and the Public Interest: Professional Power, Altruism and Alternative Medicine.* Routledge, London

Saks M (1996) From quackery to complementary medicine: The shifting boundaries between orthodox and unorthodox medical knowledge. In: Cant S, Sharma U, eds. *Complementary and Alternative Medicines: Knowledge in Practice.* Free Association Books, London

Saks M (1997a) Alternative therapies: Are they holistic? *Complementary Therapies in Nursing and Midwifery* **3**: 4–8.

Saks M (1997b) East meets West: The emergence of an holistic tradition. In: Porter R, ed. *Medicine: A History of Healing.* Ivy Press, London

Saks M (1998) Professionalism and health care. In: Field D, Taylor S, eds. *Sociological Perspectives on Health Care.* Blackwell Science, Oxford

Saks M (1999) The wheel turns? Professionalisation and alternative medicine in Britain. *J Interprofessional Care* **13**: 129–38

Saks M (2000) Medicine and counter culture. In: Cooter R, Pickstone J, eds. *Medicine in the Twentieth Century.* Harwood Academic Publishers, Amsterdam

Sharma U (1995) *Complementary Medicine Today: Practitioners and Patients.* Revised edn. Routledge, London

Stevens R (1966) *Medical Practice in Modern England.* Yale University Press, New Haven

Townsend P, Whitehead M, Davidson N (1992) *Inequalities in Health: The Black Report and the Health Divide.* 2nd edn. Penguin Books, Harmondsworth

Vincent J (1992) Self-help groups and health care in contemporary Britain. In: Saks M, ed. *Alternative Medicine in Britain.* Oxford University Press, Oxford

Witz A (1992) *Professions and Patriarchy.* Routledge, London

4

Primary care

James Dooher and Richard Byrt

There are generally considered to be three phases of healthcare activity that are fundamental to the provision of all health-related work: primary, secondary and tertiary care. These divisions are inextricably linked in terms of both concept and process, and provide the framework for health care in Britain. Primary care relates to the active promotion of a healthy lifestyle, and the continuous maintenance of health and welfare for people living in the community. It is the philosophy upon which mental health care in the community policies have been based, and has driven the closure of large institutions. Secondary care is designed to address existing health problems and includes the care of those whose primary health care needs have already been met. Tertiary care deals with optimising independence within the confines of an existing disability. This includes continuing or long stay care, many aspects of residential and nursing care and prolonged hospital care. Although these compartmentalisations provide structure they do allow some overlap where a patient may receive a single type or combination of services. Primary care can be seen as a mixed economy of care, with some services being provided free of charge, while others are not. For example, the consultation given by a general practitioner (GP) is free, but the prescription or sick note may not be. Likewise, many dentists offer both private and national health care for the same patient within the same surgery. When discussing primary care, the term patient seems to be used rather than client, customer or service user.

Many authors, including Armstrong (1998) and Baggott (1998), suggest that until relatively recently primary care has been overlooked in terms of its value to the provision of health in the UK. When we consider the range of professionals involved including GPs, community nurses, dentists, pharmacists, counsellors and midwives, and the public's universal reliance upon their services, this is rather surprising. The rejuvenated interest in primary care has been influenced by the development of the *NHS Plan* which predicted that, 'a new system of earned autonomy will devolve power from the Government to the local health service as modernisation takes hold'.

This shakedown of the NHS has produced radical reforms for the primary care sector and provides a subject for debate in all healthcare disciplines. The modernisation has been driven by a raft of reports, white and green papers, acts of parliament and latterly research. The constant within this complex world is ill health and our need to access restorative health care through self-help or professional intervention. This chapter will consider some of the complex issues which have influenced these developments.

The concept of health is both difficult to define and measure, due to its complexity and the variations in perception from cultural, gender, age, social class and location perspectives. A person who enjoys good health is said to be free from disease, enjoys a state of well-being and vigour, and is able to make appropriate adjustments to the changing circumstances of life. According to Kelly (1955, 1963) and Houston (1998) individuals function as 'active scientists', striving to make sense of their world and continually testing and revising their hypotheses about social reality. An individual's ability to relate to their world and particularly their health status, revolves around the personal constructs that they derive from an active interpretation of their world. He suggested that constructs are personal discriminations that an individual makes about situations, events and people. It is with this in mind that the simple or broad definitions of health become less valuable in truly encapsulating its meaning to the individual. An early attempt by the World Health Organization considered health to be: a state of complete physical, mental and social well-being and not merely the absence of disease or infirmity. Although this is a good effort, it fails to include the perceptions of the patient and the context in which it occurs.

Many authors have attempted to create some sort of hierarchy of need from which good health is derived. In the late 1940s, Grundy suggested a six-point scale for health and happiness which included:

- a sense of security within the family and the community
- adequate self-expression and satisfaction in personal and social activities
- affection and love, especially in infancy and childhood
- an adequate family life or some substitute for it
- an adequate and adjusted community life
- a consistent attitude towards life, a sense of purpose and a sense of responsibility to self and community (Grundy, 1949).

Maslow went on to define his hierarchy of needs in which he proposed that we are subject to two sets of motivational forces; those which ensure survival by satisfying basic physical needs and those which enable the person to realise their full potential, including intellectual and creative drives, becoming 'everything that one is capable of becoming' (Maslow, 1972). He categorised them into physiological needs, safety needs, love and belongingness, esteem needs, cognitive needs, aesthetic needs and self-actualisation. He proposed that the needs lower down the hierarchy must be accomplished before the individual can move to the next stage, with self-actualisation being at the apex of his pyramid.

There are clearly some universal givens in attempting to predict good health which go beyond simple life expectancy. But, if this is the end (pun intended), then the means must include a balance between exercise and rest, sufficient and healthy diet, intellectual stimulation, good housing and sanitary services, healthy and safe working conditions and the ability to access and use leisure facilities. Bringing these factors together to produce a meaningful nationwide strategy for health proved difficult at best. The plethora of Government advice on public health was perhaps best encapsulated by the document, *The Health of the Nation* (DoH, 1991), in which it set out the inter-relationship between its own departments including: environment, transport, education, employment and science, social security, trade and industry, agriculture, fisheries and food, with the objective of providing a cohesive and unified strategy to improve the nation's health. The particular targets were to improve national statistics with regard to:

Coronary heart disease	Pregnancy and child care
Stroke	Diabetes
Cancer	Mental health
Smoking	Communicable diseases
Eating and drinking	Physical rehabilitation
Accidents	Asthma

Through this document the Government attempted to define the priorities in health for England, and provide health care and other health-related professionals realistic targets on which to spend their finite resources. More recently, the *NHS Plan* (DoH, 2000) suggested that despite some improvements, the NHS suffers from a plethora of shortcomings that continue to undermine the quality of care it provides. These included:

- a lack of national standards
- old-fashioned demarcations between staff and barriers between services
- a lack of clear incentives and levers to improve performance
- over-centralisation and disempowered patients.

These observations were derived from public consultation which highlighted the importance for:

- more and better paid staff using new ways of working
- reduced waiting times and high quality care centred on patients
- improvements in local hospitals and surgeries.

The *NHS Plan* suggested that the NHS must be redesigned around the needs of the patient. Local services delivered and monitored locally will serve the public better than any centralised service. It predicted a new relationship between the Department of Health and the NHS to enshrine the trust that patients have in front-line staff.

The front line of primary health

The environment or setting in which health care takes place is often seen as a defining characteristic for primary care. Professionals work in buildings such as dental or doctors' surgeries, clinics, healthcare centres, or the patient's own home. The practice of primary care often takes place on a one-to-one basis between the patient and the professional. This factor creates a veil over the ability to analyse the quality of the relationship between patient and health worker. Quantitative statistics can measure the numbers of appointments, non-attendances, drug budgets and a range of hard data. It is much more difficult to assess the level and impact of patient participation. Patients want to be involved in their own care. They want to have a say in the way that their local services are developed (DoH, 2001, p. 2). The *NHS Plan* goes on to suggest that the NHS must be shaped around the needs and convenience of the patient, not the other way round; patients must have more say in their own treatment and more influence over the way that the NHS works.

In a study by Cape (2000), the findings indicated that the patient's perception of the interactions or therapeutic alliance between themselves and their general practitioner during consultations reduced symptom severity throughout the following three months. He described the significance of developing a positive and collaborative relationship as a key indicator in the treatment of emotional problems. Perceptions were based upon the listening skills of the GP, the patient's perception of the doctor's empathy and the time-span of the consultation, together with the patients own involvement in their care. All these factors were considered to be indicative of a better prognosis than if they were omitted from the interactions within a consultation. Despite the occasional research paper or case study, what actually goes on behind the surgery doors, and within the confidential confines of the doctor/patient relationship is a mystery. The intangible aspects of the relationship, such as empathy, warmth or genuineness offered by the professional are not open to public scrutiny. We can monitor the use of drugs (perhaps more for financial reasons than for any other); following the case of Harold Shipman we can scrutinise death rates, referrals to other professionals and general patient statistics, but the nature of interaction is largely unknown. The quality of the relationship between the patient and their health advisor has been further interpreted to include the development of the NHS Direct service in 1999. This is a twenty-four-hour health advice line whereby a person with symptoms can seek advice and information from the nurse at the other end of the line.

Despite the fact that primary care represents over 36% of total NHS spending (NHS Executive, 1996), it relies heavily upon the informal care of relatives and neighbours to sustain its existence, and without which it could not exist. This is not without some cost, particularly to the health of informal care. Stress is said to alter negatively our response to vaccines. Stressed care givers show poorer immune functioning and their wounds take longer to heal and they have a 63% higher mortality rate than non care-giving controls (Jones, 2000). Traditionally, the interests of patients were represented with community health councils which are being replaced by the establishment of independent patient councils in every NHS trust, including primary care trusts (PCTs).

The development of primary care walk-in centres is seen as a much needed improvement for those seeking immediate support, information and treatment, and is one of a range of responsive measures set in place. They were announced by the Prime Minister, Tony Blair on 13 April, 1999. These nurse-led centres will provide a 'drop-in' service for their local population, and provide a key role in the delivery of services, including opening hours which meet patient needs, eg. early mornings, later evening access and open at weekends. Walk-in centres are situated in a convenient location to enable easy access, cater for minor treatments, healthy lifestyle and general health information together with self-help advice to the public. They will provide a useful addition to the services offered by GPs, and although still in the pilot stage (around forty pilot centres were established during 1999/00) it is anticipated that they will provide a convenient, responsive and flexible service. The Government's optimism came under fire from the consumer body 'Which?' who conducted a series of bogus patient attendances at walk-in centres. The results were debated in the *Nursing Times* (2000; Mathieson, 2000), where claims that walk-in centres were inconsistent, incompetent and 'an extraordinary waste of staff and resources' were disputed. They cited visits to eight walk-in centres where researchers, posing as legitimate patients, presented symptoms to test the system. This covert method was considered to be unethical, and lacking in credibility. The integrity of the study was undermined by the small sample size and its undercover nature, but it did raise a serious issue about consistency and quality in the new generation of primary care facilities.

Overall, the changes have been broadly acclaimed from all quarters. Primary care professionals, such as pharmacists working in the community, are trying to develop their professional role but feel constrained by a remunerative system that is based largely on the dispensing process. The Government's agenda will provide the opportunity to move the profession forward in primary care (DoH, 2000).

On July 24, 2000 the British Association of Medical Managers produced a press release which wholly commended the developments: they suggested that the energy, enthusiasm and commitment of people who care for patients, are the focus of attention in tomorrow's NHS, following the implementation of the *NHS Plan*.

Clinical governance

The primary care agenda has been driven by a raft of Government papers, legislation and advice for good and best practice (DoH, 1996; 1997; 1999; 1999a). Central to this is the concept of clinical governance. This is a framework through which NHS organisations are accountable for continuously improving the quality of their services and safeguarding high standards of care by creating an environment in which excellence in clinical care will flourish.

There are five principle components of clinical governance:

- clear lines of responsibility and accountability for the overall quality of clinical care
- a comprehensive programme of quality improvement systems (including clinical audit, supporting and applying evidence-based practice, implementing clinical standards and guidelines, workforce planning and development)
- education and training plans
- clear policies aimed at managing risk
- integrated procedures for all professional groups to identify and remedy poor performance.

Clinical governance is a multidisciplinary/multi-agency framework designed to assist teams to provide the best possible care within their given resources. It is suggested that clinical governance will help to identify poor performance and, in part, tackle issues that cause poor performance.

The new NHS — modern, dependable (DoH, 1997) proposed that every NHS organisation is charged with the duty of embracing 'clinical governance' with quality at the core, both of the organisation and of each member of staff as individual professionals. It suggested that to facilitate this there would need to be a range of organisational changes, including the establishment of primary care groups and trusts. McCargo (2001) suggested that, 'the introduction of clinical governance could be viewed as the most radical part of the latest reforms — or indeed any of the reforms since the birth of the NHS'. This is the first time that chief executives have had a statutory responsibility for quality. It is also the first time that professional self-regulation has been seriously challenged and asked to demonstrate its ability to deliver safe care systematically and maintain public confidence.

The government suggests several benchmarks for quality, including:

❖ Professionals should be knowledgeable about the conditions that are present in primary care and skilled in their treatment and in contributing to their prevention.

❖ Professionals should be knowledgeable about the people to whom they are offering services.

❖ Services should be co-ordinated with professionals aware of each others' contributions, with inter-professional working and with no service gaps.

❖ Premises and facilities should be of good standard and fit for their purposes, and equipment should be up-to-date, well-maintained and safe to use.

The organisation of primary care: primary care groups and trusts

The Government's commitment to provide accessible and convenient services for patients which guarantee uniformly high standards saw the introduction of groups (PCGs) and latterly primary care trusts (PCTs). PCGs are the first phase of establishing the professionals involved and demonstrating that they can work together to meet the agenda and function at what is described as level one or two, which means that their work and performance is overseen by their local health authority. PCGs are governed by PCG boards which are committees of the parent health authority. The composition of PCGs generally consists of four to seven GPs, one to two community or practice nurses, one social services representative, one lay member, one health authority non-executive director and one chief executive with the chair of the board being selected from the board members.

At level one, PCGs act in support of the health authority in commissioning care for its population, and provide an advisory function. At level two they take devolved responsibility for managing the budget for health care in their area, and act as part of the health authority. The three primary tasks of PCGs are:

❖ To improve the health of, and address health inequalities in their communities.

❖ To develop primary care and community services across the primary care group.

❖ To advise on, or commission directly, a range of hospital services for patients within their area which appropriately meets patients' needs.

In England on 1 April 1999, 481 PCGs went 'live', 87% of which were operating at level two. At this time, all GPs, practice and community nurses became part of a PCG.

Once their ability has been established, primary care groups may move into a level three primary care trust and become freestanding bodies, accountable to the health authority who can then commission services. To be able both to commission and to provide services the PCT must move to what is described as a level four PCT. These PCTs are freestanding statutory bodies who undertake many of the functions of local health authorities and can run community hospitals, community health services, employ staff and own property. They are charged with the responsibility of integrating services around the needs of patients, addressing the causes of ill-health and reducing inequalities in access to services.

The intention of PCGs and PCTs is to bring together primary care professionals from both health and social care sectors, including GPs, community nurses, social workers, midwives, health visitors, pharmacists and dentists, to name but a few, who are considered to be at the front line of health advice or treatment. Together, with patient representatives and other users of their service, they take on responsibility for the healthcare needs of their local community. Because the services are being organised and delivered locally this was felt to enable greater flexibility in the provision of a quality service and provide best value for money within finite resources. The advantages of these developments suggest that PCTs will:

- put primary care professionals in the driving seat
- increase public accountability
- increase public involvement
- improve probity.

This is achieved by bringing together health and social care professionals, and other organisations and agencies working in partnership to bring about improvements in primary and community care. This will enable more responsive, dependable and integrated services which are underpinned by investment and technology, thus tackling health inequalities and delivering improvements in the quality and efficiency of patient services. The Government plan to invest one billion pounds in the refurbishment of three thousand rundown and out of date premises (DoH, 2001). Decision-making processes will be improved and it is anticipated that patients will have better access to health and social care professionals who benefit from better support and increased resources.

With forty PCTs coming into being between April and October and the existence of 434 PCGs, together with the assumption that the majority of the 130 plus prospective PCT proposals become operational from 1 April, 2001 the future of primary care is assured.

Health action zones (HAZs)

In tandem with the development of primary care groups and primary care trusts, we have seen the introduction of the health action zone (HAZ). Because HAZs work within existing structures to achieve their aims they embrace PCGs as an integral part of their structure. This initiative was first announced by the then Secretary of State for Health, Frank Dobson, in a speech to the NHS Confederation on 25 June, 1997. He proposed that the aim of HAZs was:

> ... to target a special effort on a number of areas where we believe the health of local people can be improved by better integrated arrangements for treatment and care.

His intention was to address the healthcare deficits in some of the most deprived areas in the country. Health action zones provide a long-term (seven-year) programme, which will modernise and reduce health inequalities in these areas. Mr Dobson suggested that HAZs present an opportunity to develop public involvement in ways which go beyond the traditional mechanistic approaches of formal consultation, and that they should develop to cover the whole scope of a local health improvement programme (HImP). They have three strategic objectives:

- identifying and addressing the health needs of the local area
- modernising services
- developing partnerships.

These partnerships are considered fundamental to the operation of a HAZ where public involvement is seen as a key underpinning element, integrating community initiated proposals and community governance in order to underpin local decision-making for health.

This has seen the development of assessment and planning strategies that are owned by local communities which work together in equal partnership with statutory bodies.

Conclusion

Primary care in the future should offer a more responsive and flexible system, which has in part been designed by patients for patients, with strong leadership from professionals who are more directly accountable to the recipients of their service. Fairness, equity, partnership and participation are the buzz-words, but the credibility of these goals has yet to be proven. Patients, their carers and other service users will need to become more aware of their rights, and the mechanisms to seek redress if the comfort of the *status quo* is to be challenged. Workers in primary care will need to overcome the legacy of the purchaser/provider split, bury their differences and concentrate upon delivering the stated objectives, rather than perpetuating petty power struggles in an attempt to uphold their own power base.

Key points

- ⌘ The most recent shakedown of the NHS has produced radical reforms. Some of these seem to be rejuvenated policies from the past, however, most have ensured that primary care is at the top of the health agenda.

- ⌘ The responsibilities for primary care are the same responsibilities as for public health. As public health demands grow, resources become increasingly diluted, eventually producing a solution of homeopathic proportions.

- ⌘ Front-line primary care has remained an inconsistent service. This is despite Government efforts to create a seamless uniform system, because while it offers variety, choice and quality at a good price, this is perhaps not at the same time and is dependent on the geographical area in which it is being delivered.

- ⌘ Government calls for partnership in the delivery of health will see increased devolution of the organisation, management and responsibilities of care to the general public.

- ⌘ Objectives to increase public accountability put primary care professionals in the driving seat. Increased public involvement and improved probity will ensure the future of participation and, more generally, empowerment in the choice and delivery of services.

References

Armstrong E (1998) The Primary/Secondary Care Interface. In: Brooker C, Repper J, eds. (1998) *Serious Mental Health Problems in the Community: Policy, practice and research*. Baillière Tindall, London

Baggott (1998) *Health and Healthcare in Britain*. Macmillan Press, London.

Cape J (2000) Patient related therapeutic relationship and outcome in general practitioner treatment of psychological problems. *Br J Clin Psychol* **39**(4): 383–95

Department of Health (1988) *Working Together: Securing a Quality Workforce for the NHS*. DoH, London

Department of Health (1991) *The Health of the Nation: a consultative document for health in England*. DoH, London

Department of Health (1996) *Consultation Counts. Guidelines for service purchasers and users and carers based on the experience of the national user and carer group*. DoH, London

Department of Health (1997) *The new NHS — modern, dependable*. DoH, London

Department of Health (1999) *Making a Difference Strengthening the nursing, midwifery and health visiting contribution to health and healthcare*. DoH, London

Department of Health (2000) *NHS Plan: A plan for investment, a plan to reform*. The Stationery Office, London

Department of Health (2001) *NHS Plan — An Action Guide for Nurses Midwives and Health Visitors*. DoH, London

Grundy F (1949) *The New Public Health. An Introduction to personal health and welfare services*. HK Lewis and Co, London

Houston J (1998) *Making Sense with offenders: Personal constructs, therapy and change*. Wiley, Chichester

Jones F (2000) Translating social support into health. *Psychologist* **13**(6): 296

Kelly GA (1955) *The Psychology of Personal Constructs*. Norton, New York

Kelly GA (1963) *A Theory of Personality: The psychology of personal constructs*. Norton, New York

Maslow A (1962) *Towards a Psychology of Being*. Van Nostrand, London

Maslow A (1972) *The Farther Reaches of Human Nature*. Viking Press, New York

Mathieson A (2000) Critical survey neither credible or ethical. *Nurs Times* **97**(3): 3

McCargo C (2001) Clinical governance and practice development. In: Clark A, Dooher J, Fowler J, eds. *The Handbook of Practice Development*. Quay Books, Mark Allen Publishing Limited, Dinton, Salisbury

National Health Service Executive (1996) *Primary Care: The future*. HMSO, London

NT Reporter (2000) Walk-in centres branded a waste of money. *Nurs Times* **97**(2): 6

5

The empowerment imperative in health promotion

Keith Tones and Jackie Green

The notion of health has always been contested. The concept of health promotion is also subject to multiple interpretations. For many people, for example, it is synonymous with health education. At the time of writing in the UK there is increasing debate about its relationship with public health and public health medicine and, in some quarters, a preference to redefine it as 'health development'. Traditionally, the purpose of health promotion and its predecessor health education, has been viewed unequivocally as that of enhancing public health, but under the aegis and control of public health medicine. The nature of the challenge to this traditional perspective is illustrated by a recent statement by the current Minister of Health, Alan Milburn. In a presentation at the London School of Economics he asserted:

> *'Public health', understood as the epidemiological analysis of the patterns and causes of population health and ill health, gets confused with 'public health' understood as population-level health promotion, which in turn gets confused with 'public health' understood as public health professionals trained in medicine. So by a series of definitional sleights of hand, the argument runs that the health of the population should be mainly improved by population-level health promotion and prevention, which in turn is best delivered, or at least overseen and managed, by medical consultants in public health. The time has come to abandon this lazy thinking and occupational protectionism.*

(Milburn, 2000)

This thinking reflects a general tendency to accept a broader definition of health which goes beyond the absence of disease, to include positive well-being; to move away from a narrow focus on preventive medicine; to recognise that any attempt to promote public health requires consideration of the social, cultural and economic determinants of health. This holistic perspective is increasingly accompanied by a commitment to engage actively with, and change those social and environmental structures that impose limits to health development. Such an approach is entirely consonant with the goals of empowerment that we will be examining in this chapter. We will, accordingly, describe an empowerment model of health promotion, and argue that such a model is not only consonant with the broad goals of the new public health outlined above, but also provides the most effective framework for achieving the goals of preventive medicine.

Health and its determinants

If health promotion is about promoting health, then we must have a robust understanding of the determinants of health before we can develop strategies for enhancing individual and population health status. A discussion of its elusive nature is, of course, not possible in this relatively short chapter. We will therefore merely echo the World Health Organization's now almost hackneyed assertion that health is more than the absence of disease and infirmity but a 'positive' state involving mental and social as well as physical dimensions (WHO, 1946). For our present purpose, we will accept that health has both a preventive medical dimension and also, a more holistic aspect related to well-being and the achievement of important life goals unrelated to disease. Both these dimensions, however, have many common determinants. One of the simpler and most popular representations of these influences on health appears in the 'Lalonde Report' (1974). Health (and disease), it was argued, are due to an interaction between genetic, lifestyle and environmental factors, together with the quality and availability of health services. A more sophisticated version of this analysis is in *Figure 5.1*.

Figure 5.1 describes three levels of influence. The macro level indicates the effect of national or international policies (or lack of them) on individuals' and community health, in respect of material and cultural circumstances. It would include, for example, over-arching general influences such as the extent of poverty and inequality in a nation or, more specifically, the existence of a national ban on tobacco advertising. The meso level refers to the potential effects of organisations such as local authorities, schools, hospitals or work-places: it also refers to the extent to which community norms are conducive to health or disease. At the micro level, genetic and constitutional factors clearly make a significant contribution to health, together with the influence of family and 'significant others' and individual behaviour and lifestyle. The various levels are, of course, not independent — for instance, lifestyle factors are substantially influenced by macro and meso level circumstances.

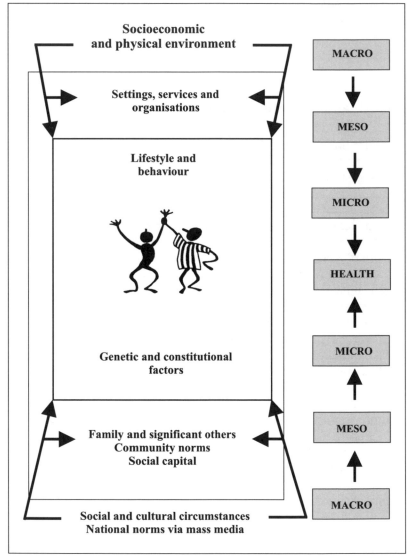

Figure 5.1: Macro, meso and micro influences on health

The concept of empowerment: individuals, communities and the environment

Like health, empowerment is an elusive concept. It can be viewed as a significant goal in its own right or, alternatively, as a means to an end. Like social justice and equity, with which it is associated, a state of empowerment may be considered synonymous with individual and social health: an autonomous individual capable of making choices is a healthy individual; an empowered community is a healthy community. In contrast, from an instrumental perspective, empowered people are assumed to be in a better position to overcome barriers and make healthy choices, for example, to resist pressures to smoke, persevere with rehabilitation programmes or exert political pressure on the local council to improve the housing stock. The World Health Organization (WHO) is quite clearly committed to empowerment. A key principle of the Ottawa Charter (WHO, 1986) asserts the importance of fostering '**active participating communities**' and has defined the main purpose of health promotion as being to help people 'gain control over their lives and their health'. For further discussion of the 'philosophical' and 'instrumental' justifications for the empowerment imperative, see Tones (1998a, b).

Essentially, empowerment has to do with the location of power — and power should reside with the people! Provided that the empowerment of communities and individuals does not militate against other people's rights to empowerment, individuals should be free to choose.

Unfortunately, free choices often prove illusory; a fact that was nicely illustrated by the late Schultz's Charlie Brown a few years ago. In this cartoon, we see Charlie Brown, who has had an uncharacteristic rush of blood to the head. He holds a snowball in his hand and faces the child virago, Lucy. Lucy looks him firmly in the eye and says, sternly, 'You may choose to throw that snowball at me. Now if you throw the snowball, I will pound you right into the ground. If you do not throw the snowball, your head will be spared.' Charlie Brown is left on his own, still holding the snowball. He contemplates the departing Lucy and muses thus, 'Life is full of choices. The trouble is you never get any!'

There are, in short, two kinds of barrier limiting choice: the first of these derives from an individual's personal characteristics and attributes; the second, and more important, is the nature of the environment, in which individuals live and work. The **actual** status and power of the individual in relation to the environment, operates at the interface between psychological characteristics of the individual and the environment in which (s)he lives and works (*Figure 5.2*).

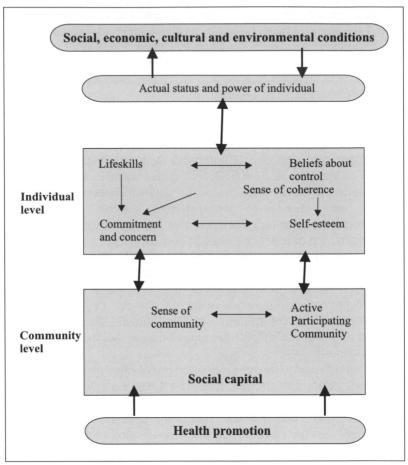

Figure 5.2: Health promotion and empowered choice (Tones, 2001)

At the core of *Figure 5.2*'s representation of the empowerment function of health promotion, is Social Learning Theory's simple but invaluable principle of 'reciprocal determinism'. On the one hand, the extent to which individuals have sufficient power to make genuine, free choices will depend on the nature of their social, economic, cultural and material circumstances. On the other hand, individuals are usually in a position to influence these environmental factors to a greater or lesser extent. Clearly, some individuals are overwhelmed by oppressive circumstances and, effectively, have no real choice. Conversely, other individuals enjoy favourable environmental conditions that facilitate choice.

Health promotion has a two-fold purpose. As many recent government initiatives designed to tackle inequality have acknowledged, the most significant — and difficult — goal is to reduce 'external' barriers to empowered choice and to develop what the Ottawa Charter describes as 'supportive environments'. The second major goal of health promotion should be to build the capacities of individuals so that they are better able to gain control over their environments at macro, meso and micro levels, even those that are relatively oppressive. The nature and dynamics of communities is increasingly considered to be important in tackling environmental obstacles to making empowered choices and in empowering individuals. Indeed, the Ottawa Charter affirmed that an 'active empowered community' was an essential prerequisite for effective health promotion. A community is, of course, more than a mere collection of individuals but is characterised by a sense of its own identity and purpose, together with a set of potentially supportive interpersonal networks. Members of an empowered community work vigorously together to tackle issues that they perceive to be a threat to their health. The ultimate manifestation of a community taking responsibility for the collective health of its members would be to challenge health inequalities. The term 'social capital' is now often used to describe empowered communities. Putnam (1995), the researcher and theorist most commonly associated with the concept, argues that:

> *'Social capital' refers to features of social organization such as networks, norms and social trust that facilitate coordination and cooperation for mutual benefit.*

> *Social capital... foster[s], '... sturdy norms of generalized reciprocity'... Facilitate[s] coordination and communication, amplif[ies] reputations,and thus allow[s] dilemmas of collective action to be resolved... [Moreover,] dense networks of interaction probably broaden the participants' sense of self, developing the 'I' into the 'we'... enhancing the participants' taste for collective benefits.*

> (Cooper *et al*, 1999, p. 7, quoting Putnam, 1995)

There is a two-way relationship between community and individual levels. An empowered community will also generate empowered individuals: empowered individuals will contribute to increasing the stock of social capital. Both together will maximise the chances of engaging effectively with, and gaining control over, the social, economic and material environment. Success breeds more success and institutes a 'virtuous circle'.

Self-empowerment and related notions

Turning now to the individual level, the attributes of self-empowerment have been thoroughly documented and researched. Some of these attributes are represented in *Figure 5.2*. Essentially, an empowered individual has, in relatively high measure, a number of key beliefs and skills, together with positive feelings related to those beliefs and skills. Beliefs about control are at the heart of self-empowerment and associated feelings of well-being. They indicate the extent to which people can actually exercise control (though of course, beliefs about control and actual control are not one and the same, since it is possible to believe that you are in control of situations when you are not, and vice versa!). At one end of a kind of continuum of control, we can identify '**cognitive control**', where individuals understand what is happening or about to happen to them, even though they actually have no real control over events (for example, understanding what will happen in a surgical procedure and what it will feel like after the event). '**Behavioural control**', however, occupies a position further along this continuum: the individual now has the knowledge and skills to exercise some control over events (for instance, has learned how to control pain by breathing appropriately or asking for pain killers). The notion of '**perceived locus of control**' (PLC) may be located at the opposite end of the continuum. PLC refers to a **generalised** belief about control, ie. the belief that by and large whatever happens in life — good or bad — is substantially due to individual actions and capabilities. Rotter (1966) initially described this generalised belief system. He used the term '**internal**' locus of control to describe those people who believed that in general, and by and large, whatever happened to them in their lives was the result of their own efforts and competences. In contrast, those governed by an '**external**' locus of control, believe that their lives are controlled by chance, fate and/or powerful others. Research suggests that 'internals' are more likely to adopt health-promoting behaviours than externals. We should also note at this point, the similarity between extreme externality and the pathological state described by Seligman (1975) as 'learned helplessness'. This condition is the very antithesis of self-empowerment and Seligman argued convincingly that six major symptoms of learned helplessness had almost exact parallels in clinical depression.

It will be noted in *Figure 5.2* that beliefs about control contribute to self-esteem. The desirability of a realistically-based, relatively high level of self-esteem would almost certainly be generally accepted. Apart from the mental health aspects, those having a high level of self-esteem would seem to be better able to resist unwanted social pressures and be more inclined to 'look after themselves'. Again, this affective dimension would seem to be located at the opposite end of the empowerment spectrum from learned helplessness.

The importance of one further control belief must be particularly emphasised. This is the belief that Bandura (1977; 1982) defined as 'self-efficacy'. It is simple but essential and is best illustrated in the context of another 'formula' derived from Social Learning Theory, represented as follows:

$$\text{response efficacy} \times \text{self-efficacy} = \text{action}$$

Briefly, individuals are likely to adopt a healthy course of action (or indeed, any course of action) to the extent that they believe that the action will result in some significant benefit for them (ie. 'response efficacy'), and also that they are actually capable of performing that action. For instance, heavy smokers may well believe that they would benefit from giving up, but do not even attempt to do so because they are convinced, due to previous failures, that they could not possibly succeed in the endeavour.

It is worth observing in passing that a number of other psychological constructs are related to self-empowerment. Probably the most relevant of these was described by Antonovsky (1979) as a 'sense of coherence'. This concept is central to Antonovsky's 'salutogenic' approach to health, with its emphasis on positive, holistic health outcomes. The approach, in Antonovsky's words is 'negentropic', ie. well-being and control is associated with making sense out of chaos. This in turn results from a sense of coherence, defined by Antonovsky as, 'a global orientation that expresses the extent to which one has a pervasive, enduring though dynamic feeling of confidence that one's internal and external environments are predictable and that there is a high probability that things will work out as well as can reasonably be expected' (Antonovsky, 1979, p. 123).

A sense of coherence has three main components:

❖ Comprehensibility: the world is believed to be 'ordered, consistent, structured and clear... and the future predictable' rather than 'noisy, chaotic, disordered, random, accidental and unpredictable'.

❖ Manageability: individuals believe that they have the kinds of resources at their disposal which will enable them to manage their lives.

❖ Meaningfulness: life makes sense emotionally; people are committed; they invest energy in worthwhile goals.

It will be apparent that 'comprehensibility' and 'manageability' are both entirely consistent with the other empowering beliefs and capabilities mentioned above. However, we should emphasise the point that it is perfectly possible for individuals to be convinced that they do not have control over their lives (perhaps because of illness or religious convictions) but, on the other hand, to feel that life is meaningful. In terms of positive mental health and engagement with life, the meaningful dimension will frequently compensate for beliefs about lack of control.

Before leaving our review of a sense of coherence, it is seen in *Figure 5.2* that 'commitment and concern' have been included as part of individual level empowerment. To be accurate, these constructs — as, indeed, meaningfulness more generally — would not be included in the usual catalogue of empowerment characteristics. However, meaningfulness is central to Antonovsky's con-ceptualisation of coherence and it certainly makes an essential contribution to acting on behalf of others in an 'active empowered community'.

One final point must be made about self-empowerment, and this has to do with the role of 'life skills'. The term life skills refers to a set of learned capabilities, that help individuals cope with and gain control over life circumstances. A full discussion is not possible here (see Tones [1994] for a more complete review). They include, for example, skills in managing stress, making decisions, being assertive and working effectively in groups. As readers' own experience will confirm, it is often remarkably difficult to influence people's efficacy beliefs (and even more difficult to convert 'externals' into 'internals'); any amount of persuasion and exhortation is likely to have little effect. The solution to the problem is encapsulated in the gnomic observation that 'nothing succeeds like success'.

How to ensure success? One effective strategy centres on the technique popularised by Social Learning Theory: modelling. If an individual observes a model with whom he or she identifies (ie. one sharing similar circumstances, characteristics and predicaments), succeeds in a particular task (eg. taking recommended, graduated exercise after a coronary or stroke or successfully breast-feeding a child), then that individual is likely to believe that (s)he is capable of achieving the same goal (assuming of course that (s)he really wants to). Not infrequently, the desired activities cannot be carried out without the acquisition of particular competences: for instance, heavy drinkers who have seen the error of their ways may not believe that they would be capable of resisting social pressures to join in the round-buying culture at the bar. They are doubtless right, and observing a model operate successfully would probably be insufficient in itself. It would also be necessary to provide opportunities to learn a number of verbal and non-verbal assertiveness skills, together with the opportunity for practice and gaining feedback on performance. In other words, education for health and life skills is a key component of empowerment in the situation described above.

Before giving more consideration to the process of empowerment at macro, meso and micro levels, we should at this juncture, be clear about just what is involved in the essentially contested notion of health promotion, and offer a model for practice based on empowerment principles.

An empowerment model of health promotion

We have already noted current difficulties in defining health promotion. We feel that it is reasonable to consider that the purpose of health promotion is to improve the health of the public and its essence is encapsulated in the simple 'formula':

health promotion = health education x healthy public policy

It is often said that it is difficult to define policy but easy to recognise it. As Cunningham (cited in Ham and Hill, 1985, p.11) put it:

> *'Policy' is rather like the elephant — you recognise it when you see it but cannot easily define it.*

It is concerned with the exercise of politics and the practice of power is at its very core. 'Healthy public policy' — to use the terminology of the Ottawa Charter — is, therefore, concerned to achieve health goals by essentially political means, involving the development and implementation of fiscal and economic measures designed to bring about environmental change at macro, meso and micro levels. A whole range of policies will impact on health — hence the call for 'health impact appraisal', ie. accountability in all areas of policy for health impact (WHO, 1988). Health education can be defined with more precision and certainty:

> *Health education is any intentional activity which is designed to achieve health or illness related learning, ie. some relatively permanent change in an individual's capability or disposition. Effective health education may, thus, produce changes in knowledge and understanding or ways of thinking; it may influence or clarify values; it may bring about some shift in belief or attitude; it may facilitate the acquisition of skills; it may even bring about changes in behaviour or lifestyle.*

> (Tones and Tilford, 1994, p. 11)

The interaction of these two broad modes of intervention, policy and education, is summarised in *Figure 5.3*. Unlike preventive approaches to health promotion, where the sole concern is to coerce people into health (often in an authoritarian fashion), *Figure 5.3* describes an empowerment model.

Promoting healthy public policy

First of all, health should be viewed in accordance with the classic WHO definition, ie. not just the prevention and management of disease, but also a positive state relating to quality of life and well-being (including empowerment itself as a desirable healthy endpoint).

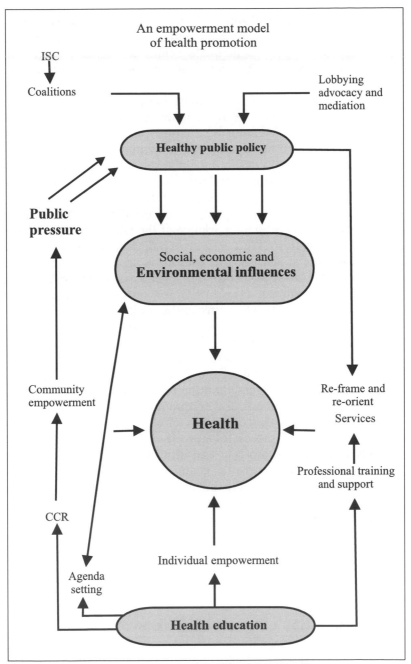

Figure 5.3: An empowerment model of health promotion

We can observe from *Figure 5.3* that 'healthy public policy' is mobilised in order to influence those social, economic and environmental factors that facilitate health and militate against ill health. Major political factors that traditionally influence the development and implementation of policy are categorised in terms of lobbying and advocacy (by individuals and powerful organisations). Advocacy is considered to be lobbying by the powerful on behalf of the relatively weak. Mediation (again a term derived from the Ottawa Charter) refers to the fact that compromise may have to be reached between different and conflicting interests, such as health versus profit. *Figure 5.3* also acknowledges one of the most important strategies for exerting pressure on policy development — coalitions of the great and the good. Again, coalitions involve collaborative working with partners, in the parlance of the Ottawa Charter, 'inter sectoral collaboration' (ISC). Effective collaboration is notoriously difficult to achieve and, for this reason, is separately signalled in *Figure 5.3*. The Boise Project provides a good example of an effective coalition (see Goodman *et al*, 1993 for further examples). This particular initiative aimed to improve the health of older people in a US city in Idaho. A non profit-making health promotion research centre acted as a lead agency and created a coalition of local employers, Boise School District, YMCA and YWCA, the State university, two local hospitals, the District Health Department, the Idaho State Office on Ageing and the Idaho Division of Health. As with all effective coalitions, the community itself was involved; in this specific example, the community of elderly people. The project achieved a range of successful outcomes, not only in respect of changes in individual lifestyle and attitudes but also in effecting policy change. For instance, changes were made in various organisations catering for the needs of elderly people in Boise, including the regional medical centre. At the macro level, the city and state increased financial support for older people. Furthermore, the initiative was disseminated to other states and similar programmes were sponsored in over 100 communities in thirty states nation-wide (Kemper and Mettler, 1990).

The contribution of health education

It should be noted that the function of health education envisaged in *Figure 5.3* differs from its traditional, so-called victim-blaming concern with persuading individuals to adopt behaviours that would lead to the prevention of disease. Health educators retain their role of working with individuals and groups. However, their prime concern is not with persuasion, but with empowering choice by building individual and group capacities and seeking to remove or minimise obstacles to those choices.

Health education also has a major contribution to make in relation to training and advice for those working in the various health services. The 'new' health education would be concerned with the 'reorientation of health services' (again, to use a term from the Ottawa Charter); for example, health promoters would want to ensure that the strategies and methods used by organisations, such as schools, workplaces and hospitals, were consistent with the empowerment philosophy. Furthermore, a highly significant goal for health educators is to contribute to a 'reframing' process in order to create awareness that services such as transport, housing, and economic development actually contribute to health and may have a greater impact (for good or ill) than the medical services proper.

The most radical function of the 'new health education' is one of raising critical consciousness about public health needs. The term 'critical consciousness' is derived from Freire's (1974) work in adult education; its purpose is not just to raise awareness but to generate indignation about social pathogens, such as inequality and inequity and mobilise community action. Community empowerment and the creation of social capital are part of this process. Clearly, it can be argued that community empowerment is a health goal in its own right, but an effective empowerment process should also result in mounting public pressure on those holding the reins of power at government or local level. The endpoint would be the creation of 'healthy public policy'.

One especially important educational strategy for creating critical consciousness and policy change is now generally described as 'media advocacy'. In short, the most valuable function of mass media is viewed not as persuading individuals to adopt healthier lifestyles but rather, to generate critical consciousness. A discussion of this strategy, together with an 'A to Z' of other advocacy and lobbying techniques, will be found in Chapman and Lupton (1994).

The term 'agenda setting' is included in *Figure 5.3*. This is a diluted form of media advocacy, in that it places health issues on the public agenda (rather than striving more actively to create pressure for change). It is often used by governments when contemplating new policy measures (perhaps in the form of a carefully planned 'leak' to journalists) in order to be sure that the policy in question will not result in electoral unpopularity. In contrast, genuine media advocacy will often address policy issues which a given government would never choose to implement.

Action at macro and meso level

A full discussion of examples of the many potential varieties of empowerment in action is not possible here. We will merely draw attention to the work of such campaigning organisations as ASH (Action on Smoking and Health) which, over the years, has raised awareness of the iniquities of the tobacco industry and made a substantial contribution to the development of policy banning tobacco advertising. Empowerment at the meso level is best illustrated by reference to such settings as 'health promoting' schools, workplaces and, of course, the 'health promoting hospital'. Currently in the UK, a number of less formal, *ad hoc* initiatives — such as 'health action zones' and 'healthy living centres' — have been established for the purpose of empowering communities and addressing the continuing problem of inequalities in health. We will illustrate meso level empowerment by referring to the 'health promoting hospital'.

The health promoting hospital

The roots of a 'settings approach' to health promotion are to be found in WHO's development of the 'healthy cities' movement. In short, a setting is more than a geographical location, such as a school, in which to deliver health education. The setting is viewed as a whole system, in which all aspects of an organisation's functioning and ethos is consistent with achieving healthy outcomes. For instance, a school should not just address issues such as self-esteem in personal, social and health education lessons, but should also ensure that all aspects of school life foster self-respect. To the extent that empowerment is both a healthy goal in its own right and, at the same time, a means of increasing the likelihood of individuals making healthy choices, then any health promoting setting should incorporate a whole system strategy consistent with empowering all those in that organisation.

A major impetus for the establishment of health promoting

hospitals was the Budapest Declaration (WHO, 1991). The suggestion that the hospital should be concerned with promoting health as well as curing disease was regarded in some quarters as bizarre; to then suggest that hospitals should be concerned with empowerment was risible! However, Goffman's (1961) classic definition of the hospital as a prime example of a 'total institution' supported the common sense view that hospitals tended to depersonalise and actually disempower patients. Taylor (1979) also noted that the hospital was one of the few places where the individual forfeits control over virtually every task he or she customarily performs. She went on to observe that patients adjusted to this exercise in disempowerment by becoming either 'good patients' (who slavishly and subserviently complied with staff demands) or 'bad patients' who rebelled against this authoritarian regime. Nonetheless, many hospitals have, in fact, joined the network and made real efforts to meet the criteria for WHO recognition. Key criteria relating to empowerment can be summarised as follows:

- there should be a focus on health rather than on disease (empowerment is intrinsically healthy)
- patients and their relatives should be the beneficiaries of good communication and sound health education
- there should be a concerted effort to empower actively patients (and staff)
- the hospital should be 'outward-looking' and establish a 'healthy alliance' with its community.

(Tones, 1993)

It is doubtless obvious that the creation of health promoting hospitals involves often major policy and organisational changes that militate against years of tradition and professional socialisation. The problem of medical dominance will doubtless strike a chord with all those who have worked in a hospital setting. On the other hand, an empowering strategy explicitly acknowledges the complementary roles of all who work in the setting. In relation to nursing, Macleod Clark (1993) has called for a shift from what she calls 'sick nursing' to 'health nursing'. She categorises these as follows:

Sick nursing: dominating, generalised, prescriptive, reassuring, directive.
Health nursing: collaborative, individualised, negotiated, supportive, facilitative.

(Macleod Clark, *ibid*, p. 260)

This description of 'health nursing' is evidently consistent with an empowering strategy 'at the micro level'.

Empowerment at the micro level

At first glance, it might seem that empowerment requires major organisational and political change. Given that the fundamental barriers to empowerment are inequity and inequality, this is not an unreasonable assumption. However, individuals working with other individuals can and do contribute to empowerment — often in small but significant ways.

It is, for instance, possible to identify quite clearly the processes and components involved in a successful empowering encounter between, say, a nurse and a client or patient. Many of these processes have already been described and researched quite extensively, for example, in work on behaviour modification, motivational interviewing and non-directive client counselling.

Before commenting on the major features of an empowering encounter, it is important to note that the organisational culture and environment can militate against operating in an empowering way when face-to-face with a patient or client. For instance, Wilson-Barnett and Latter (1993) demonstrate how successful empowerment of patients at ward level is associated with the empowerment of the nurses themselves. As the authors argue:

> *The ward climate needs to be such that nurses feel valued, supported, autonomous and empowered members of the ward team. This appeared to facilitate health education and health promotion via increasing morale and enabling nurses to support and empower their patients rather than maintain traditional role distinctions and the unequal balance of power inherent in these. ... [The] empowerment of nurses was closely associated with a democratic management style from the ward sister... a flattened ward hierarchy and devolved decision-making.*

(Wilson-Barnett and Latter, 1993, pp. 68–69)

The components of an effective empowering encounter are summarised below.

Components of an empowering encounter

❖ Establish rapport using social interaction skills such as active listening and demonstration of empathy; (simply listening to somebody enhances their sense of worth and is empowering).

❖ Explore existing felt needs, beliefs and feelings about the matter under discussion. (For example, failure to take account of clients' 'theory' of their illness probably makes a substantial contribution to the typical 50% 'non compliance' rate.)

❖ Explore the client's environment and circumstances. Look for barriers to the implementation of the desired outcomes.

❖ Gain the client's agreement to a course of action that is jointly agreed (establish a 'contract').

❖ Provide appropriate supportive education,eg. in addition to supplying information, influence efficacy beliefs, using modelling where appropriate; provide any necessary skills.

❖ Provide support, eg. opportunity to become a member of a support group; ensuring that clients receive benefits to which they are entitled; look for ways to contribute to environmental change; lobbying housing agencies on their behalf.

❖ Since substantial change requires substantial measures outwith the control of individual health workers, act as an advocate — both as an individual and through membership of professional bodies — for the implementation of healthy public policy.

However, it would be wrong to assume that the adoption of empowering strategies, even in a small way at the face-to-face level, is easy. Furthermore, any assumption that this happens all the time as part of routine professional practice would be misguided. For instance, Kendall's (1993) revealing study of the ways in which health visitors communicated with mothers of children about nutrition showed that even the 'nursing process' — trained health visitors (whom Kendall thought should have known better!) tended to talk a lot, rarely listened and frequently failed to take account of the beliefs, attitudes and existing dietary practice of the mothers. As Kendall put it:

> *... it appears that health visitors need to develop facilitative skills which will elicit and promote client participation. Clients cannot be expected to be actively involved in and comply with healthcare recommendations if they are not being acknowledged as equals and their own experiences*

and perspectives being taken into account... [health visitors'] apparent need to control clients rather than negotiate with them must be confronted and tackled both at the educational and practice levels...

(Kendall, 1993, p. 116)

It would, of course, be unreasonable to expect that all the tasks and roles previously outlined could be achieved by one individual. Different members of a team have different skills, competencies and access to resources and it is worth reiterating the fact that an empowering health promoting setting should provide an opportunity for teamwork and collaborative working.

Key points

- ⌘ There have been many interpretations of 'health promotion', with recent emphasis on community action to change social, cultural and economic factors affecting health.

- ⌘ A model of influences on health is proposed. These include the interaction of: the total socioeconomic and physical environment; health service and other organisations; community norms; family and other significant people; genetic and constitutional factors; and individual lifestyle and behaviour.

- ⌘ Empowerment can be viewed both 'as a significant goal in its own right' and as a means of achieving a desired aim, in relation both to individuals and to whole communities. Empowerment is concerned with 'the location of power'. Individual and environmental factors, and their inter-relationship affect empowered choice.

- ⌘ The World Health Organization has emphasised fostering 'active participating communities'; and has stated that the chief aim of health promotion is enabling individuals to 'gain control over their lives and health'. This can be achieved at different levels.

- ⌘ Empowered communities have aspects of social organisation ('social capital') which facilitate participation. Such communities generate empowered individuals and vice versa. An empowering model of health promotion is concerned to influence both individual empowerment and changes in wider society through community action and political activity.

❋ Empowered individuals believe they have control over things that happen to them. Beliefs about control, including self-efficacy, contribute to individuals' self-esteem and the extent that they engage in healthy behaviours. Also relevant to psychological empowerment is the individual's 'sense of coherence': belief in the predictability of the environment, and that life is manageable and meaningful. The acquisition of 'life skills' may help individuals 'gain control over life circumstances'.

❋ 'Healthy public policy' is concerned with changing social factors which adversely affect health. This is achieved through advocacy, mediation, and coalitions between various organisations, with participation of community members. The 'new health education' aims to be empowering, and to raise 'critical consciousness about public health needs', eg. through the skilful use of the media.

❋ Examples of empowering initiatives include health-promoting hospitals and schools that aim to promote health through all aspects of organisational life. Health-promoting hospitals enable patients to maintain control. The organisational cultures and environments of health services, and the extent that nurses feel valued, can influence the empowerment of service users.

❋ 'Components of an empowering encounter' include 'active listening and empathy'; taking account of the client's perspective, circumstances and environment; jointly agreed action; and providing support, education and advocacy.

References

Antonovsky A (1979) *Health, Stress and Coping*. Jossey-Bass, San Francisco

Bandura A (1977) Self efficacy: toward a unifying theory of behavioural change. *Psychol Rev* **64**(2): 191–215

Bandura A (1982) Self-efficacy mechanism in human agency. *Am Psychologist* **37**(2): 122–47

Chapman S, Lupton D (1994) *The Fight for the Public Health: Principles and Practice of Media Advocacy*. BMJ Publications, London

Cooper H, Arber S, Fee L, Ginn J (1999) *The influence of social support and social capital on health: A review and analysis of British data*. Health Education Authority, London

Cunningham C (1985) In: Ham C, Hill M, eds. *The Policy Making Process in the Modern Capitalist State*. Wheatsheaf, Brighton

Freire P (1974) *Education and the Practice of Freedom*. Writers and Readers Publishing Cooperative, London (originally published in Portuguese, 1967)

Goffman E (1961) *Asylums. Essays on the social situation of mental patients and others*. Doubleday, New York

Goodman RM, Burdine JN, Meehan E, McLeroy KR (1993) Special issue on community coalitions. *Health Education Research: Theory and Practice* **8**(3): 122–31

Kemper DW, Mettler M (1990) Building a positive image of ageing: the experience of a small American city. In: Bracht N, ed. *Health Promotion at the Community Level.* Sage, Newbury Park

Kendall S (1993) Client participation in health promotion encounters with health visitors. In: Wilson-Barnett J, Macleod Clark J, eds. *Research in Health Promotion and Nursing.* Macmillan, London

Lalonde M (1974) *A New Perspective on the Health of Canadians.* Government of Canada, Ottawa

Macleod Clark J (1993) From sick nursing to health nursing: evolution or revolution? In Wilson-Barnett J, Macleod Clark J, eds. *Research in Health Promotion and Nursing.* Macmillan, London

Milburn A (2000) *Health and Economics.* Speech at the London School of Economics, 8th May, 2000

Putnam RD (1995) *The strange disappearance of civic America.* The American Prospect No. 24, downloaded pages 1–17. Online at: http//:www.putn.html

Rotter JB (1966) Generalized expectancies for internal versus external control of reinforcement. *Psychological Monographs* **80**(1): 1–28.

Seligman MEP (1975) *Helplessness: On Depression, Development and Death.* WH Freeman, New York

Taylor SE (1979) Hospital patient behavior: reactance, helplessness, or control? *J Social Issues* **35**(1): 156–84

Tones BK (1993) The theory of health promotion: implications for nursing. In Wilson-Barnett J, Macleod Clark J, eds. *Research in Health Promotion and Nursing.* Macmillan, London

Tones BK (1994) Health promotion, empowerment and action competence. In: Jensen B, Schnack K, eds. *Action and Action Competences.* Royal Danish School of Educational Studies, Copenhagen

Tones BK (1998a) Health education and the promotion of health: seeking wisely to empower. In: Kendall S, ed. *Health and Empowerment: Research and Practice.* Arnold, London

Tones BK(1998b). Empowerment for health: the challenge. In: Kendall S, ed. *Health and Empowerment: Research and Practice.* Arnold, London

Tones BK (2001) Health promotion, health education and the public health. In: Dettels F, McEwen J, Beaglehole R, Tanaka H, eds. *Oxford Textbook of Public Health.* 4th edn. Oxford University Press, Oxford

Tones BK, Tilford S (1994) *Health Education: Effectiveness, Efficiency and Equity.* 2nd edn. Chapman Hall, London

Tones BK, Tilford S (2001) *Health Promotion: Effectiveness, Efficiency and Equity.* 3rd edn. Thornes Nelson, London

Wilson-Barnett J, Latter S (1993) Factors influencing nurses' health education and health promotion practice in acute ward areas. In: Wilson-Barnett J, Macleod Clark J, eds. *Research in Health Promotion and Nursing.* Macmillan, London

World Health Organization (1946) *Constitution.* WHO, Geneva

World Health Organization (1986) *Ottawa Charter for Health Promotion. An International Conference on Health Promotion,* November 17–21. WHO, Copenhagen

World Health Organization (1988) *The Adelaide Recommendations. Healthy Public Policy.* WHO/EURO, Copenhagen

World Health Organization (1991) *The Budapest Declaration on Health-Promoting Hospitals. Business Meeting on Health Promoting Hospitals, 31 May–1 June, 1991.* WHO, Copenhagen

6

User participation and empowerment in community mental health nursing practice

Jayne Breeze

Introduction

Empowerment has been defined as giving power or authority, giving ability, enabling, and permitting (McLeod, 1987). It has been contended elsewhere that empowerment is, in reality, a complex subject encompassing a diversity of needs and agendas (Morgan, 1993) and is best understood by the effects of its absence: 'powerlessness, helplessness, hopelessness, alienation, victimisation, subordination, oppression, paternalism, loss of a sense of control over one's life' (Gibson, 1991, p. 355).

The last decade has seen a substantial move towards empowering the users of mental health services in the United Kingdom through the promotion of choice and shared decision making. This concept underpins government legislation (DoH, 1998) and has been a focus of debate among the nursing profession (Gibson, 1991; Skelton, 1994). Paradoxically, however, the pressure on community mental health nurses to ensure that people with serious mental health problems comply with treatment, especially medication, has never been greater (Gardner *et al*, 1999).

Given this dichotomy, it is unsurprising that it is contended that some mental health workers, including nurses, place a low priority upon user participation and some actively do not want it at all (Campbell and Lindow, 1997). Nevertheless, studies have consistently identified that service users want more choice and control in care delivery (Rogers *et al*, 1993; Shepherd *et al*, 1994; Seymour, 1998; Breeze and Repper, 1998; Goodwin *et al*, 1999). It is important that user participation and empowerment are analysed within the context of community mental health nursing practice.

This chapter aims to do this by assessing the evidence of empowerment in practice and the dilemmas this creates, addressing the relationship of power to the concept of empowerment; and, finally, suggesting changes that community mental health nurses can bring to their practice which promote greater choice and control for the service user.

Means and Smith (1994) identified three main strategies for achieving empowerment. These are:

- empowerment through 'exit'
- empowerment through 'voice'
- empowerment through 'rights'.

This provides a useful framework for examining empowerment in relation to community mental health nursing practice.

Empowerment through 'exit'

The empowerment strategy of 'exit' is a means of enabling the user to have choice between services with the option of 'exiting' from one service, that is, choosing another, if dissatisfied (Taylor *et al*, 1992). This was a strategy particularly favoured by the Conservative administration of the early nineteen eighties, who sought to empower service users by replacing the monopolistic provision by the public sector with an internal market system that utilised a mixed economy approach. It was asserted that 'promoting choice and independence underlies all the Government's proposals' (DoH, 1989, p. 4).

The viability of this strategy was questioned in relation to how real this was for people with long-term disabilities or health problems, given that many are living on low incomes, thus limiting their choice within the independent sector (Means and Smith, 1994). In addition, empowerment through 'exit' neglects the point that factors other than choice often determine the use of mental health services (Onyett, 1992).

The current Government's reform of the NHS Act (DoH, 1997) has committed to replacing the internal market with integrated care. In addition, the opportunity to exit from mental health services is further threatened with the introduction of compulsory community treatment orders as proposed by current mental health policy (DoH, 1998), to be used as one means of increasing compliance with treatment. Many organisations representing users and providers of mental health services (including the Community Psychiatric Nursing Association) criticise this move and argue that there are alternative methods to achieve compliance that are as effective as compulsory treatment orders, but also maintain autonomy and dignity (MIND, 1999).

One alternative that has gathered momentum is that of assertive outreach, which is a form of intensive case management based upon the 'assertive community treatment' model used in the USA. It is contended that it is of particular benefit for people with multiple and complex mental health needs, who are traditionally difficult to engage and therefore often 'non-compliant' (Seymour, 1998). As this method is dependent upon the relationship between worker and user, it is viewed as empowering, especially when compared with compulsory treatment. The components of an empowering relationship being: respect; empathetic understanding; and choice and flexibility (Repper *et al*, 1994; Morgan, 1996; Perkins and Repper, 1996; Breeze and Repper, 1998).

Some commentators caution against the unquestioning implementation of assertive outreach, arguing that the USA's model changed from a supportive system that focused upon developing users' strengths and independence to one that prioritised treatment compliance from which it was almost impossible to 'exit' (Smith *et al*, 1999). However, it has been observed that supporters of assertive outreach in the UK are just as concerned that this should not happen (Freeman, 2000). The intensive case management model that assertive outreach is based upon certainly advocates that community case managers should focus upon service users' strengths and aspirations, while enabling the user to set her/his own agenda (Onyett, 1992; Repper *et al*, 1994).

What all parties appear to agree on is the central importance of developing a worker-client relationship that enables the service user to have equal participation in decision making. This would put the emphasis upon alliance rather than compliance (Perkins and Repper, 1998) and should involve the service user choosing from a range of skilled interventions (Gardner *et al*, 1999; Perkins and Repper, 1996). The opportunity of choice would enable him/her to 'exit' one type of intervention in preference to another.

This is reliant upon the service user receiving the appropriate information in order to make an informed choice. However, some choices may be viewed as harmful and, when seen to be made for irrational reasons or due to lack of competency, pose dilemmas for community nurses. Many would find it difficult not to intervene under such conditions, creating a conflict between respect for autonomy and duty of care.

However, the assessment of rationality can be based upon value judgements (Breeze, 1998). In addition, what is seen to be a decision to 'exit', based upon irrational reasons, may have actually followed a careful weighing up of the costs and benefits of continuing with the treatment (Perkins and Repper, 1998). For example, a person with serious and long-term mental health problems may prefer to live with the consequences of relapse, rather than endure the side-effects of medication.

Nevertheless, the community mental health nurse may need to enter the 'grey area of compromise', in order to address the conflict of individual rights versus duty of care (Perkins and Repper, 1998). Given these ethical dilemmas, as well as the current and proposed legislative and policy framework for mental health service delivery, the strategy of empowerment through 'exit' has limitations. This is particularly the case for people with multiple and complex needs, who may pose a risk to themselves or others.

Empowerment through 'voice'

One means of addressing the problems of empowerment through 'exit' is the promotion of empowerment through 'voice' (Hoyes *et al*, 1993). This also enables service users to change aspects of a service that they are otherwise happy with and do not wish to exit (Taylor *et al*, 1992). It seems especially important for users who are unable to exit a service or for whom exit would entail a high cost (Means and Smith, 1994). Also, people's experiences as inpatients can sometimes be traumatic and community mental health nurses can empower service users by listening to their accounts and taking them seriously (Lindow, 1996; Campbell and Lindow, 1997).

The emphasis on obtaining users' views when conducting health service research is a relatively recent phenomenon. The agenda was set within government legislation at the beginning of the last decade, which determined the promotion of consumer feedback and working in partnership with service users who, it was contended, should have a central role in developing and planning their own care (DoH, 1991). This occurred in parallel with health professionals beginning to acknowledge the importance of the user's perspective (DoH, 1994), and is now firmly entrenched in mental health care policy (DoH, 1998).

While seeking the user's view appears to have gathered momentum over the last decade, it has usually been done by means of client satisfaction surveys (Goodwin *et al*, 1999). However, such questionnaires leave little room for people to express their own view about the subject in hand since all the items are usually predetermined as standardised items by the researcher (Rogers *et al*, 1993). Earlier studies have also highlighted the limitation in using this approach. Kaufman *et al* (1979) attempted to synthesise the interests of both clients and professionals in order to compile a client survey instrument. They found that there was disagreement between clients and professionals as to what questions were desirable. On reviewing the literature, Ridgeway (1988) found that people who have experienced mental health problems, and the people who provide services to them, often see the world from very different perspectives. This can be overcome by ensuring that there is opportunity for subjective accounts and the freedom of self-expression (Rogers *et al*, 1993; Strauss, 1994).

An example of this method of examining the user's perspective on care can be found in a small study which focused upon service users, perceived by mental health nurses to be 'difficult' to care for, due to their multiple and complex needs and challenging behaviour (Breeze and Repper, 1998). A major theme throughout the study was that of power and control. This is not surprising, as it is a common theme within many user-focused studies (Rogers *et al*, 1993; Shepherd *et al*, 1994; Seymour, 1998; Goodwin *et al*, 1999). What is worthy of note is that people who are difficult to engage or work with, without exception, recount experiences of having no control over their care (Breeze and Repper, 1998; Seymour, 1998) whereas the generic studies indicate a mixed picture.

Control is manifested in different ways that is either directly observable (such as forced treatment, threats or coercion) or less tangible (such as withholding information, lack of involvement in care planning). The first experience of this lack of control is encountered on admission to hospital; where neither did the respondents want to be, nor did they feel that they had any control over the admission. Being a 'voluntary' patient appeared not to change this feeling, 'I was given a choice, either come in voluntarily or get detained. I knew I had to come in' (Breeze and Repper, 1998, p. 1303).

Once in hospital, some of the respondents found their movement restricted and their behaviour curtailed. They often referred to their environment in terms of its being a prison. For example, the secure ward on which some respondents spent part of their admission due to high risk behaviour was referred to as 'the lock up', while one respondent described restriction on movement as, 'it was like, it was sort of being in a prison and then sometimes not even let out in the exercise yard' (Breeze and Repper, 1998, p. 1305). This view of hospital as prison was also prevalent in the study by Goodwin *et al*, (1999) and is a comparison that has been presented by Foucault (1971).

A common theme throughout studies that focus upon the users' perspective appears to be experiences of forced treatment, particularly medication. This was certainly a prominent feature within the Breeze and Repper study. When persuasion did not work ('come on, they'll do you good') then direct threats often followed: 'Well they said you've got a choice, you either, you can either take it orally or if not, you'll be physically restrained and given an injection, and I didn't want an injection so...' (Breeze and Repper, 1998, p. 1305). Only one respondent recounted experience of negotiating a nursing care plan, yet research has indicated that service users wish to have greater input into decision making (Shepherd *et al*, 1994).

A more subtle means of control appeared to be exerted through the restriction on the service users' 'voice'. Examples of this were lack of access to clinical meetings (eg. ward rounds), 'tokenistic' attendance at care programming meetings ('Well, it's all really cut and dried anyway, you know, its all been decided already', Breeze and Repper, 1998, p. 1306), and not being believed or taken seriously. While it has been identified that service users' and professionals' priorities differ (Shepherd *et al*, 1994), Breeze and Repper (1998) found that when this occurred professional priorities always took precedence, dismissing the concerns of the service users.

All the respondents acknowledged responding to restriction, forced treatment and being ignored with challenging behaviour, incurring self-harm, aggression to others or 'absconding'. That is, there appeared to be increasing struggles for control.

In keeping with other studies (Rogers *et al*, 1993; Seymour 1998; Goodwin *et al*, 1999) the service users identified positive aspects of care as: being treated with respect, essentially as a person, but, more than that, as a valued person (for example, through staff exuding warmth, displaying empathy); being enabled to have some meaningful control over their care; and being listened to and, especially, being believed (Breeze and Repper, 1998). These characteristics can be considered as components of empowerment (Hokanson Hawks, 1991). In keeping with Goodwin *et al* (1999), the respondents valued the nurses making time to be with them and, as identified by Rogers *et al* (1993), they also valued 'ordinary contact' and 'normal' conversations.

Nevertheless, while these aspects are considered of value to a positive care experience, this does not appear to be enough. Service users who are difficult to engage or be cared for, also identify **skilled** intervention as being an important factor (Breeze and Repper, 1998; Seymour, 1998).

Even the caring nurses — some are better at it than others, you know, you can be a caring nurse and still be crap. They still care but they haven't got the expertise to get it out of you, you know, what's up with you.

(Breeze and Repper, 1998, p. 1307)

In order that mechanisms for 'voice' actually lead to empowerment, the changes that service users ask for should be taken on board by community mental health nurses. This may be in relation to their own practice or negotiating with colleagues within inpatient facilities. The consistency with which some grievances appear in studies focusing upon the user views, for example, lack of information regarding diagnosis and treatment (Rogers *et al*, 1993; Breeze and Repper, 1998; Goodwin *et al*, 1999), suggests that more needs to be done if tokenism is to be avoided.

Empowerment through 'rights'

Throughout the eighties and early nineties, Government perception of empowerment through the strategy of 'rights' was viewed as being essentially about individuals having the right to pursue their own goals, objectives and to meet their own needs, free from intrusive state intervention (de Jasey, 1991). This position was in opposition to many in the disability movement who argued that this view is meaningless for the majority of service users who exist on low incomes and who argue for a rights-based approach to cash (Means and Smith, 1994). Certainly, research has indicated that service users' main concerns are generally economic, eg. with regard to housing, benefits, etc (Shepperd, 1994).

The current Government appears to have adopted a more interventionist approach and believe that mental health service users have the right to expect care provision to be 'safe, sound and supportive' (DoH, 1998). Empowerment through 'rights' should not only address the right to refuse treatment but also should acknowledge the right to access the appropriate support and care when in distress (Perkins and Repper, 1998). Research has found that community mental health services can be withdrawn from people because of their disturbed or disturbing behaviours (Repper and Perkins, 1995).

Activists within the disability movement argue that policies should aim to minimise the avoidable disadvantages while compensating for others, in order to equalise life chances for all (Coote, 1992). This appears to have been taken on board in the Disability Discrimination Act 1995. Beresford *et al* (1996) draw parallels between having a physical disability and being a user or survivor of the mental health system, especially from a civil rights perspective. Both groups of people experience oppression and discrimination in employment, housing, education, social situations and in personal relationships. They argue that the common ground for people with physical disability and people with mental health problems is that they are disabled by the lack of appropriate social and personal support.

Civil rights are often fought for by protest and collective action, but are dependent upon this culminating in changes to legislation to promote these rights and protect them in law. It could be argued that despite progress being made by, for example, the Disability Discrimination Act (1995), there is still a long way to go before people with mental health problems and social disability achieve equality.

Concept of empowerment

Whichever strategy is adopted, most would agree that empowerment involves service users taking, or being given, more power, which implicitly involves taking at least some power away from providers (Means and Smith, 1994). A necessary condition for empowerment, is the willingness (or ability) of health workers, eg. nurses, to relinquish the need for control (Labonte, 1989). For this to happen, nurses themselves must be empowered (Chavasse, 1992). Skelton (1994) challenges this assumption, arguing that there is no evidence to suggest that once empowered, nurses would then share this power with users. Nevertheless, one study found that nurses who were 'powerful' were more likely to empower service users than the nurses considered to be powerless (Raatikainen, 1994). However, there were no significant differences between the two groups in relation to 'difficult' patients, which suggests that the empowerment of people with multiple and complex mental health problems may be more complicated. The behaviour of 'difficult' patients can often engender feelings of 'powerlessness' in nurses (Carey *et al*, 1990).

In addition, nurses may feel pressured into controlling patient behaviour because of organisational pressure (Porter, 1993). These aspects were mirrored by a mental health nurses' focus group discussion considering the phenomenon of patients who present challenges (Breeze and Repper, 1998). The findings from this study suggested that threats to the nurses' competence and control were important factors when defining patients as 'difficult':

> *We have to have a controlling environment — the reason I think we control is because if we don't control something we feel out of control.*

> (Breeze, 1997)

As many of the service users considered within the focus group were detained under a section of the Mental Health Act 1983, the nurses generally felt obliged to 'take control' even if this incurred a struggle. They felt that they would be letting other patients down if they did not attempt to control disruptive behaviour.

This can be mirrored in the community where disruptive behaviour can create pressure for the nurse to intervene to protect the public. Community mental health nurses can feel 'powerless' when service users are difficult to engage or refuse to comply with treatment (Seymour, 1998). Breeze and Repper (1998) also found that the nurses were more likely to feel challenged when they were short staffed than when resources were perceived to be adequate. Organisational pressure to 'move people on quickly' was seen as creating the frustration when patients did not respond to nursing intervention.

This struggle for control by nurses, as well as service users, implies that empowerment is not a linear process but is more complex. This may be because control in this sense can be better explained by examining the concept of power. Perkins and Repper (1998) point out that the terms 'power' and 'empowerment' appear as if interchangeable within the literature. They argue that while empowerment is a psychological concept, felt within an individual, power is political, referring to structural conditions and power relationships between groups and individuals.

Power

The concept of power is complex and the plethora of literature on the subject fails to produce a single, uniform conceptualisation of the term (Cavanaugh, 1984), and there appears to be little agreement as to whether it is intentional, structural or both (Abercrombie *et al*, 1988).

Power as agency is essentially, behavioural as it involves a person or group of people having power over another person or group of people (Stevens, 1983). This would suggest that the action is intentional and within the control of the dominant agents (ie. the holders of power). When applied to service users' accounts of having no control over their care, it would suggest that this was due to intentional acts by the care providers. The implication is that the power lies at the hands of the dominant agents, that is, power can be given not taken. This could explain how service users are only able to have any control over their care when professionals have been prepared to give it. However, it does not explain why nurses can feel powerless or why service users can be perceived as a threat to their control.

An alternative view that addresses these problems is that power is predominantly structural (Layder, 1985). The emphasis within the notion of structure is that social relations are ongoing, organised, and relatively enduring, that is, reproduced social relations transpose and influence individual agency. Many structural theorists appear to argue that structural power inherently involves conflict between the oppressor and the oppressed. This would explain how nurses could perceive themselves to be powerless as they can see themselves as 'victims' of the organisation too; as involuntary detainment and organisational power can be positioned within the context of 'an ongoing set of reproduced relations'.

Flaws in this theory can be observed when it is applied to service users' accounts of their experience with mental health nursing practice. Firstly, it does not account for the power differentials between nurses and the service users. That is, it can be contended that however powerless nurses are within the mental health system, they are more powerful than the service users. Secondly, it does not account for the differences in approaches within the nursing staff. While studies present accounts of enforced care, there appear to be other examples where users have been given some control and choice.

This would suggest that there are limitations to viewing power solely in terms of either agency or structure. Steven Lukes (1974) attempted to resolve this 'structure versus agency' problem by offering a 'radical view' of power as an alternative. He contended that other theorists tended to stop at a 'one-dimensional' or 'two-dimensional' view of power. Lukes claims that his view is radical because it contains a third dimension.

Lukes (1974) sees the one-dimensional view in terms of observable decision making, indicating direct conflict concerning the subjective interests of the people involved. Examples of this are involuntary admissions, enforced care and restriction of movement or behaviour. Luke criticises the one-dimensional view by stating that it wholly focuses upon behaviour in the form of overt decision making on issues where there is an observable conflict of subjective interests. He argues that this focus does not acknowledge unobserved interests or that people may be unaware of what their interests are.

Lukes (1974) suggests that the two-dimensional view of power includes not only the overt decision making outlined above, but focuses upon non-decision making as part of the use of power. Power may be used to suppress challenges by preventing certain issues being discussed, or decisions about them being taken. This involves covert, as well as overt conflict concerning the subjective interests of individuals. Lukes, in discussing this typology of power, suggests that it can include coercion, influence, authority, force and manipulation. An example might be the situation of a community mental health service user, with serious and long-term mental health problems, who refuses to comply with medication. The often covert, yet nevertheless, underlying threat of being compulsorily admitted to hospital, may influence compliance (Szasz, 1983). There was certainly evidence of this in the study conducted by Breeze and Repper (1998).

Lukes (1974) also criticises this view of power for remaining behavioural and because it can be located, alongside the one-dimensional view of power, within the notion of power based upon agency. Lukes, therefore, adds a third dimension of power, which breaks away from this focus upon behaviour by suggesting that the manifestation of power is not reliant upon the action of individuals (or groups) but may, indeed, be manifested by inaction: that is, power can be exercised by manipulating the wishes and desires of social groups.

While the first and second-dimensional views of power require conflict (either overt or covert) to be present, in Lukes' third-dimensional view of power, he argues that 'A' can have power over 'B' without any sign of conflict; for example, just because 'B' appears to want to comply does not mean that 'A' has not got power over 'B'. A possible example of this third dimension of power within mental health practice is the legitimacy of psychiatrists to define the criteria for the term 'patient'. In keeping with Lukes' typology of the third-dimensional view of power, the absence of conflict (either overt or covert) may not necessarily mean that being defined as a 'patient' is in the 'interests' of the person with a mental health problem (see, for example, Chamberlin, 1988).

Lukes' third-dimensional view of power also enables a perspective of power in relation to service users with multiple and complex needs. The struggles for control identified within Breeze and Repper's (1998) study suggest that this group of service users are less affected by the third-dimensional view of power as proposed by Lukes (1974); and are more likely to be involved in the conflict endemic within the first two dimensions of power, which may precipitate mental health care workers defining someone as 'difficult'.

Criticism of Lukes' 'radical view' of power suggests that he has not really resolved the problem of 'agency versus structure' as he has retained the dichotomy (Giddons, 1979); and, despite his own assertions, has maintained a focus upon the behavioural aspects of power (Layder, 1985). Despite its limitations, this view of power could be used by community mental health nurses to inform their practice in relation to power and empowerment.

The notion of power and agency, and its emphasis upon individual or group behaviour, denies the constraints that nurses work under within the mental health system. It would suggest that mental health workers, as individuals, are in control of all the power they have over service users. While this may be true to a point, it does not explain how much of this power remains enduring, despite changes in personnel. The notion of power and structure, on the other hand, does not explain how individual mental health workers are able to empower or oppress, albeit within the system. For example, service users have identified that some nurses can, and do, form empowering relationships with them.

Suggestions for change

Lukes (1974) offers a framework from which community mental health nurses can effect changes to their practice in order to promote empowerment of service users, while understanding any limitations brought about by constraints from structural power. A consistent feature, throughout studies that focus upon users' views, is that service users appreciate empowering nurse-patient relationships that demonstrate respect and which enable them to have some choice and control.

Treating someone with respect includes treating that person as an equal. This can be manifested in seemingly small ways such as engaging in ordinary conversations. However, treating someone as an equal is also about acknowledging the expertise that they can bring to the care process (Perkins and Repper, 1998). While community mental health nurses have varying expertise when assessing, planning and implementing care, it will be the service user who brings with them the experience of having a mental health problem and using the mental health services. This will be expertise that few nurses have, and could form the foundation of a real partnership in care.

As previously discussed, having choice and control in relation to care and treatment is important to service users and yet, according to user accounts, this can be limited or even absent. However, while a major change in attitude may be required, this can be brought about by arguably small changes with little expense.

To have choice requires accessible and understandable information. Unfortunately, people with mental health problems may not receive this. For example, Rogers *et al* (1993) found that 60% of a sample who had received major tranquillisers reported not being informed of their purpose. While this is the medical domain, community mental health nurses can help service users to negotiate with consultant psychiatrists (Campbell and Lindow, 1997) as well as ensuring that they have access to relevant information relating to their care.

Enabling service users to have more control and choice in their care also requires that nurses **listen** to them. While listening skills are an integral part of nurse training, nurses do not always hear the needs, choices and aspirations that the service users are trying to convey. This may be because nurses, along with other mental health professionals, are focusing upon their own assessment of need and priority of goals. Sometimes service users are thought to be 'unrealistic' in what they want, when really it is the lack of resources or ingenuity of the service that is the problem (Perkins and Repper, 1996).

Enabling service users to have greater control over their care requires that they receive adequate and appropriate information, that they are listened to, and that their choices are not ignored because they do not fit with the professional view of what is important. As already discussed, community mental health nurses can feel anxious about retaining control when the person is seen as being a risk to themselves or others. They can feel a need to protect, both from a legal and a moral obligation.

However, there are identified strategies for user involvement in risk assessment that enable some choice and control (Campbell and

Lindow, 1997; Hird and Cash, 1999), including the components of empowerment already discussed. An example of such a risk assessment would contain: the service user's perspective of risk, which is often wider than that considered by professionals and includes aspects such as deprivation (Ryan, 1999); utilising strategies already undertaken by the service user to manage risk in the past; integration of the service user's expressed need and associated risk with 'normative' needs as introduced by the mental health nurse into the care plan (Hird and Cash, 1999).

Intervention may be seen to be particularly 'justified' when the person is assessed to be incompetent to make a particular decision (Breeze, 1998). There are suggested safeguards for this that enable the service user to retain some choice and control. These might include the use of a 'crisis card' to give advance directives of how she/he wishes to be treated when in a crisis situation (DoH, 1994), or an advance directive care plan on which the service user and community mental health nurse have worked together (Hird and Cash, 1999).

Perkins and Repper (1996) offer a model of working with people who have serious and long-term mental health problems that enables a practical framework of empowerment for community mental health nurses. The model, referred to as 'social disability and access', is underpinned by the following premises:

1. 'The person is central: her/his interests and preferences as well as social circumstances' (Perkins and Repper, 1996, p. 28). On helping someone to gain access to the social world, it is essential that the nurse identifies which social facilities, roles, relationships and activities the service user wishes to access. This entails listening to the service user and enables empowerment through 'voice'.

2. 'A range of different interventions, supports and strategies can be utilised' (p. 28). The service user should be able to choose, not only from a range of caring and treatment options, but from different care providers, for example, professionals, voluntary agencies or self-help organisations. This would enable empowerment through 'exit'.

3. 'The focus shifts from changing the disabled individual to changing the society' (p. 29). This involves adaptation of the social world to aid access for the socially disabled service user that parallels adaptation of the environment for people with physical disability, for example, ramps and wide doors required to give access to people with mobility problems. This highlights

the responsibility of society, rather than putting all emphasis upon the service users' skills and could be said to enable empowerment through 'rights'.

Conclusion

User participation and empowerment in community mental health nursing practice will not be easy. The constraints of structural power can render feelings of powerlessness in nurses as well as service users. As already discussed, the ethical dilemmas produced by the conflict of individual right to autonomy versus duty of care and the proposed changes in mental health law and policy, such as community treatment orders, may serve to exacerbate this feeling, especially in relation to people with multiple and complex needs. Examples of good practice within the literature suggest that, despite these constraints, empowerment of service users can be promoted.

Community mental health nurses can foster empowering relationships with service users that focus upon alliance and partnership. This involves respect, empathy, being listened to, receiving information and having meaningful choices within the care process. The central importance of this relationship to promoting user empowerment cannot be over emphasised. The typology of empowerment through 'exit', 'voice' and 'rights' (Means and Smith, 1994) can provide a useful means of examining whether user empowerment is real or tokenistic, while the model of social disability and access (Perkins and Repper, 1996) can offer a useful framework to apply this in practice.

Challenging established ways of working is not easy, especially when the change is not desired by all. However, some of the changes asked for by service users, such as being given a 'voice', could be brought about relatively easily, yet have a real impact upon how service users view their services. As has been argued elsewhere:

> *When people not used to speaking out are heard by those not used to listening, real changes can be made.*

(Beeforth *et al*, 1990, p. 16)

Thanks to Julie Repper for her comments on an earlier draft of this chapter.

The publishers and editors acknowledge, with thanks, Blackwell Science Publications for copyright permission to publish material previously published in Breeze and Repper (1998) and Breeze (1998).

Key points

- ⌘ There has been a recent dichotomy in DoH policy for mental health services, between enabling empowerment and exerting increased control. The literature suggests that, while service users want 'more choice and control in care delivery', some mental health professionals see service user participation as a low priority.
- ⌘ Empowerment through 'exit' enables the service user to leave one service for another. However, choice for some individuals is limited by low incomes, lack of information and community treatment orders. Assertive outreach has been said to involve empowering relationships; but its 'unquestioning implementation' has been criticised, particularly if it is impossible to 'exit' expectations of treatment compliance. However, nurses are faced with ethical dilemmas if they consider clients' choices to be harmful.
- ⌘ Empowerment through 'voice' enables service users to effect changes in services with which they are dissatisfied. Recent DoH policy has stressed service user views. Surveys of the satisfaction of clients generally include items which fail to take account of their perspectives. Community mental health nurses need to take on board clients' suggestions, in order to empower them.
- ⌘ In a research project, service users seen as 'difficult' described many restrictions, including 'forced treatment' following admission, with dismissal of their concerns. They appreciated being valued and respected by staff. Respondents emphasised the need for skilled nursing interventions and 'empowering nurse-patient relationships... enabling them to have... choice and control.' Clear, accessible information and listening to service users are needed. Clients' perspectives in risk assessments are important, as are plans of care, agreed in advance by service user and nurse, for implementation in periods of crisis.

⌘ The most recent Conservative governments viewed empowerment through 'rights' as freedom from State interventions. The Disability Movement argued that this had little meaning for people on limited incomes, and that rights should be related to life opportunities. More recently, New Labour policy has considered rights in relation to access to appropriate support and services.

⌘ There are conceptual limitations in viewing power only with reference to individuals and social structures. Lukes (1974) proposed, in addition, that some power does not involve overt conflict or direct action. An example is a client's decision to take medication only because of the fear of compulsory admission if (s)he does not comply. The author found that nurses felt under pressure to 'take control' when 'difficult' behaviour occurred and when there were 'organisational pressures'.

⌘ Perkins' and Repper's 'model of working with people with serious and long-term mental health problems' premises the centrality of the individual; using a variety of 'interventions, supports and strategies'; and shifting the focus 'from changing the disabled individual to changing the society.'

References

Abercrombie N, Hill S, Turner BS (1988) *The Penguin Dictionary of Sociology*. Penguin Books, London

Beeforth M, Conlan E, Field V, Hoser B, Sayce L (1990) *Whose Service is it Anyway? Users' Views on Co-ordinating Community Care*. Research and Development for Psychiatry, London

Beresford P, Gifford G, Harrison C (1996) What has disability got to do with psychiatric survivors? In: Read J, Reynolds J, eds. *Speaking Our Minds*. Macmillan Press, Basingstoke

Breeze J (1997) *The Care Experience of the 'Difficult' Patient*. Unpublished dissertation, Sheffield University, Sheffield

Breeze J (1998) Can paternalism be justified in mental health care? *J Adv Nurs* **28**(2): 260–5

Breeze J, Repper J (1998) Struggling for control: the care experiences of 'difficult' patients in mental health services. *J Adv Nurs* **28**(6): 1301–11

Campbell P, Lindow V (1997) *Changing Practice. Mental Health Nursing and User Empowerment. Royal College of Nursing, London*

Carey N, Jones SL, O'Toole AW (1990) Do you feel powerless when a patient refuses medication? *J Psychosoc Nurs* **28**(10): 19–25

Cavanaugh M (1984) A typology of social power. In: Kakabadse A, Parker C, eds. *Power, Politics and Organisations*. John Wiley and Sons, Chichester

Chamberlin J (1988) *On Our Own*. MIND Publications, London

Chavasse J (1992) New dimensions of empowerment in nursing — and challenges. *J Adv Nurs* **17**: 1–2

Coote A (1992) *The Welfare of Citizens: Developing New Social Rights*. Institute of Public Policy Research, London

de Jacey A (1991) *Choice, Contract, Consent; A Restatement of Liberalism*. Institute of Economic Affairs, London

Department of Health (1989) *Caring for People: Community Care in the Next Decade and Beyond.* DoH, London

Department of Health (1991) *The Patients' Charter.* DoH, London

Department of Health (1994) *Working in Partnership: A Collaborative Approach to Care.* DoH, London

Department of Health (1997) *The new NHS — modern, dependable.* DoH, London

Department of Health (1998) *Modernising Mental Health Services: Safe, sound and supportive. A national strategy for mental health.* DoH, London/NHSE HSC, Leeds: 1998/223

Foucault M (1971) *Madness and Civilization. A History of Insanity in the Age of Reason.* (Translated by Howard R.) Tavistock Publications, London

Freeman J (2000) Can ACT take off? *Ment Health Nurs* **20**(8): 14–16

Gardner B, Owen L, Thompson S (1999) Compliance: The need for a fresh approach. *Ment Health Nurs* **19**(5): 18–22

Gibson CH (1991) A concept analysis of empowerment. *J Adv Nurs* **16**: 354–61

Giddens A (1979) *Central Problems in Social Theory.* Macmillan, London

Goodwin I, Holmes G, Newnes C, Waltho D (1999) A qualitative analysis of the views of in-patient mental health service users. *J Ment Health* **8**(1): 43–54

Hird M, Cash K (1999) Mental health service users and risk. In: Ryan T, ed. *Managing Crisis and Risk in Mental Health Nursing.* Stanley Thornes Ltd, Cheltenham

Hokanson Hawks J (1991) Power: a concept analysis. *J Adv Nurs* **16**(6): 754–62

Hoyes L, Jeffers S, Lart R, Means R, Taylor M (1993) *User Empowerment and the Reform of Community Care: An Interim Assessment.* School for Advanced Urban Studies, Bristol

Kaufman S (1979) Synthesising the interests of consumers, citizens and administrators in gathering client feedback. Evaluating and program planning, vol 2: 263–7. Cited in: Huxley P (1990) *Effective Community Mental Health Services.* Avebury/Gower Publishing, Aldershot

Labonte R (1989) Community and professional empowerment. *Can Nurse* **85**(3): 23–8

Layder D (1985) Power, structure and agency. *J Theory of Social Behaviour* **15**: 131–49

Lindow V (1996) What we want from community psychiatric nurses. In: Read J, Reynolds J, eds. *Speaking Our Minds.* Macmillan Press, Basingstoke

Lukes S (1974) *Power: A Radical View.* Macmillan, London

McLeod W (1987) *The New Collins Dictionary and Thesaurus in One Volume.* Collins, London

Means R, Smith R (1994) *Community Care: Policy and practice.* Macmillan, London

MIND (1999) *Ten Questions About Compulsory Treatment in the Community.* MIND, London

Morgan S (1993) *Community Mental Health: Practical Approaches to Long-Term Problems.* Chapman and Hall, London

Morgan S (1996) *Helping Relationships in Mental Health.* Chapman and Hall, London

Onyett S (1992) *Case Management in Mental Health.* Chapman and Hall, London

Perkins R, Repper J (1996) *Working Alongside People With Long-Term Mental Health Problems.* Chapman and Hall, London

Perkins R, Repper J (1998) *Dilemmas in Community Mental Health Practice: Choice or Control.* Radcliffe Medical Press, Abingdon

Porter S (1993) The determinants of psychiatric nursing practice: a comparison of sociological perspectives. *J Adv Nurs* **18**: 1559–66

Raatikainen R (1994) Power or the lack of it in nursing care. *J Adv Nurs* **19**: 424–32

Repper J, Ford R, Cooke A (1994) How can nurses build trusting relationships with people who have severe and long-term mental health problems? Experiences of case managers and their clients. *J Adv Nurs* **19**: 1096–104

Repper J, Perkins R (1995) The deserving and undeserving: selectivity and progress in a community care service. *J Ment Health* **4**: 483–98

Ridgeway P (1988) *The Voice of the Consumer in Mental Health Systems: A Call for Change.* Institute for Program Development, Burlington, Vermont

Rogers A, Pilgrim D, Lacey R (1993) *Experiencing Psychiatry. Users' Views of Services.* Macmillan/MIND, Basingstoke

Ryan T, ed (1999) *Managing Crisis and Risk in Mental Health Nursing.* Stanley Thornes Ltd, Cheltenham

Seymour E (1998) *Keys to Engagement.* The Sainsbury Centre for Mental Health, London

Shepherd G, Murray A, Muijen M (1994) *Relative Values.* The Sainsbury Centre for Mental Health, London

Skelton R (1994) Nursing and empowerment: concepts and strategies. *J Adv Nurs* **19**: 415–23

Smith M, Coleman R, Allott P (1999) Assertive outreach: a step backwards. *Nurs Times* **95**(30): 46–7

Stevens K (1983) *Power and Influence*. John Wiley and Sons, New York

Strauss JS (1994) The person with schizophrenia as a person: approaches to the subjective and complex. *Br J Psychiatry* **164**(suppl 23): 103–7

Szasz T (1983) *Ideology and Insanity*. Marian Boyers, London

Taylor M, Hoyes L, Lart R, Means R (1992) *User Empowerment in Community Care*. School of Advanced Urban Studies, Bristol

7

Woman's empowerment — myth or reality

Judith Reece and Carrie White

Introduction

In the second year of a new millennium the progress of humanity is dogged by war and political unrest. The last hundred years have seen world-wide technological and lifestyle changes for most, however, despite liberalism within Euro-centric economies women in some sections of society have become increasingly disempowered.

Despite the general trend to decarcerate the residents of institutions into community facilities, the building and development of high and medium secure hospitals has increased, perhaps driven from a media feeding frenzy of high profile incidents involving people with mental health problems. Of those diagnosed with mental health problems residing in secure facilities, and those carrying a burden of a criminal conviction, women represent a very small proportion of the total population. However, at the start of the new century they remain a somewhat disempowered group. The origins of this disempowerment go back many more centuries.

While women have more freedoms than our fore-sisters ever dreamed of, there remain areas where they are still the victim. Sometimes along with men, they exist in regimes that serve only to remove any sense of power and control over their own destiny. The secure unit represents an area where caring and the exercise of professional power come together, and should empower the residents, to return to a society that saw them as a threat to its existence. We are not even convinced what the concept of empowerment means as Fraher and Limpinnian (1999, p. 147) note, 'Empowerment can be what you want it to be, depending on different agendas'.

If empowerment can be what we want it to be, the question of its existence as a tangible reality, rather than a mythological or abstract paradigm, should be considered. Is it a cherished ideal, a quoted theory or a political goal that is lost in the language of rhetoric, and perhaps is a feature of Government statements on healthcare idealism? The area of mental health care and nursing has often been asked to put the empowered client at the top of the healthcare pyramid. However, it has not achieved its goal of empowerment for all patients, especially those who are detained in a secure environment. Empowerment is a much-used concept, but it is now so value laden that it appears to have lost credibility, and professional carers speak eloquently of giving back that which they had no right to take away in the first place.

The Department of Health in 1994 stated that, 'Mental health nursing should re-examine every aspect of its policy and practice in the light of the needs of the people who use services' (p. 3). The wrongful exercise of professional power has a history as long as the healthcare system itself, and certainly predates any notion of the NHS or professional caring. Yet, as Potier noted (1993), power does not always have to be negative and controlling. Good care and a mutual approach to care, rather than professional labelling and control, can be a potent source of energising mental health. Potier states:

Power does not have to be a pejorative concept, it is energy which can be used positively to facilitate change with and for people.

(Potier, 1993, p. 338)

WISH (Women in Secure Hospitals) would support this statement.

WISH is a unique national charity working with, and on behalf of, women during, after and at risk of secure containment in high security hospitals, medium secure units and prison psychiatric units.

WISH staff seek to empower the women and build their self-esteem and confidence through the development of positive long-term relationships. WISH staff advocate on their behalf when necessary but, primarily, seek ways to support the women to voice their own needs and concerns. WISH liaises with nursing staff, clinicians, managers, social workers and off-ward services, through informal contact and formal meetings. The aim is to influence improvements in the quality and appropriateness of care that is provided for women patients. WISH is also working on a national level to change the overall legal, medical and institutional framework that places women in secure care (WISH, undated).

The experiences of women can be better understood when they are linked to the general oppression of women as a group in an unequal society, where 'there are still very distinct gender roles and expectations. Women are still predominantly expected to take the main responsibility for domestic work and child rearing. Women still dominate occupations related to domestic, menial, caring and low paid work.

> *We are still portrayed in the media as sex objects, and are still the victims of actual and potential sexual violence both in and outside the homes. Women are still expected to look pretty, speak quietly, and act gently, and if we deviate from such stereotypical behaviours we are often judged as 'bad', 'mad' or 'both'*

(Stafford, 1999, p. 3)

Men are more likely to commit persistent and random violent and sexual offences against strangers. Compared to men, very few women commit crimes, even fewer commit violent crimes. According to Home Office figures (1995) over four times as many men were found guilty or cautioned of a criminal offence, as were women. In respect of crimes involving violence against the person, men outnumbered women by over five to one (42,000 against 7,800). When women do commit violent offences, the offence is usually isolated and takes place within a clear family social context. However, the precipitating factors are rarely taken into account when sentencing women. Nor, too, are the antecedents, eg. physical, sexual and emotional abuses. Lloyd (1995) noted that in court women who have committed crimes, particularly violent crimes, are twice as likely as men to be dealt with via psychiatry: because they have stepped so far outside their approved social role, they are perceived to be 'mad'.

Over 26% of women in high security hospitals are detained on a civil order under the Mental Health Act (1983), ie. their detention is not linked to any prosecuted criminal offence. This only applies to 9% of male patients in these hospitals. Fritchie (1999) noted that, 'The routes by which women become recipients of mental health care are (in the majority of cases) different from those of male users.' Their needs are consequently also different. Fritchie went on to say:

> *The therapeutic and other needs of women patients are substantially different from those of male users of the service. Force fitting services for women into a system designed for men does a disservice to women.*

(Fritchie, 2000, p. iii)

The discriminatory process by which women are judged is dis-empowering; women are then further disempowered by the very system that purports to help them. However, the experiences of female patients in secure hospitals can mirror the oppression of women in wider society (Cowan, 1996). This is considered in the next part of this chapter which examines prevailing myths about empowerment and the role of women.

Myth 1: Pre-registration nurse education cultivates empowerment in students

The new entrant to nursing may be someone who has a great deal, or no practical experience of what it means to care for a patient. Part of that learning is gaining some sense of the history of nursing, and of the students' socialisation into that profession. It is that very process of being transformed into a professional carer, from a keen but non accountable caring friend, which is the starting and to an extent, ending point, of nursing education. Along the way, nurses learn both theory and acquire practical skills that will make them into practitioners who are 'Fit for purpose'. At the end of the process they are then assumed to be accountable practitioners who will care and be accountable for the clinical decisions they make. One of the more subtle yet constant features of the nursing education process is the oft unspoken, but present notion of elitism in caring. Nursing is not a unitary concept that can be applied wherever care is indicated. Neither for that matter are all nurses viewed in the same light by either society or each other. Nurses are very often the organisers of care, yet they have only limited power to prescribe it. They do the work of caring, may even prescribe parts of it, and yet are themselves disempowered by medicine in the professional hierarchy. However, some areas of nursing have greater 'value' than others; technological skill is highly valued and is currently closely linked with funding allocations and salary scales. It is possible to suggest that in some practice domains nurses exercise considerable power and authority. This, in itself, reinforces a degree of elitism that has beset nursing in modern times. In some situations, this has served to alienate nurses from the rest of the team and create distance between the recipient and the provider of that care (Mowforth, 1999).

We know that not all areas of nursing or nurses are the same. Some have very successfully limited this elitist power both in terms of empowering the client and in terms of creating a team of carers, rather than a mixture of competing professionals, who fight over 'their patient'. Mowforth (1999) notes that:

> *The ethos of the superior-elitism of nursing and the attendant power base needs challenging. Nurses are not a homogenous group, nor are they an isolated group within health care.*

The nursing student may experience the authoritarianism that is still inherent in many areas of healthcare training but is noticeable in both nursing and medicine. Nursing students are taught, gain experience and are assessed in the skills of delivering care to a client, sometimes, as in the case of secure provision, against the consent of the person concerned. They are given and acquire for themselves the ability to see that they 'do to' the deserving patient. The past can be replicated in patterns of training. The student enters the world of nursing with all its customs and traditions and may become as disempowered by the process as the clients they are learning to care for. They learn the language of 'the expert'. They learn the language of power and empowerment but, until very recently, were relatively powerless in changing the nature of their own learning.

Even with changes in the education process and content, the undergraduate nurse mostly has little power over the content of her/his training any more than the teachers themselves have. The teaching institutions respond to targets and skill acquisition norms that are set out for them by local and national training imperatives. While these may improve the quality of care, they do not always improve the way in which care is owned by the cared for. It remains a gamble for a student to challenge poor or dated practice. It remains a very disempowering experience to make a formal complaint; the fear of recrimination is perceived as reality even if it is just a perception. If we cannot be convinced that we are making education empowering, then can we expect students to become empowering practitioners in situations of control, where the exercise of justifiable authority can easily become an abuse of power? Maybe empowerment is a myth.

Myth 2: The acceptance of empowerment means that women are no longer oppressed

Ever since Mary Wollstonecraft spoke out for the rights of women in 1792 and probably before that, women have fought for the right to be seen as and be productive members of their society. They have wanted this in a manner that was not always related to their role in the reproduction of the species. Women have been and still are oppressed by a patriarchal society which justifies the use of male power to reinforce that control. Women still take up mental health services in greater numbers than men do. Yet, we know that for many women the source of that mental distress rests with the male. Women are still the victims of rape and assault because they are women and they still suffer mental trauma as a direct or indirect result, as is testified by the work of Herman among others. We like to think that such oppressions have ended but this is simply not the case as Herman has indicated in her work on trauma. Society still treats the woman who is a victim of violence, and who reacts against that in a variety of ways from assault on self or others in retaliation, by reasserting all too often a power based response.

> *The power of society in institutionalising and dis-*
> *empowering women, particularly through the operation of*
> *criminal justice and psychiatric institutions is far reaching.*

(Herman, 1992, p. 388)

This power can be at the institutional or personal level, and few in the total institutions of prison or secure psychiatric wards are able to work against that. If they do so as carers, then they face isolation and can be forced out all together as Potier experienced. Candib (1994) discusses the value of true feminist woman-centred empowered caring. She, like many other nursing commentators, places true empowered caring in the province of empathy. We cannot speak of empowerment in nursing care if we do not have empathy and true respect for the woman. The woman's distress has to be seen in the context of her experience of oppression. Many of us cannot easily voice this oppression, it may not always be present all the time, but for those of us who have experienced early trauma, oppression and mental vulnerability are a reality. We also need to understand that as carers, we are not immune either; there are no 'we' and 'they'.

Breeze and Repper (1998) addressed the issue that even where empowering care is presented as a standard, the struggle for control remains an issue. It is as if both sides are trying to gain therapeutic advantage over one another. It may be that future training standards for practitioners will include the attainment of the skill of enabling the rebuilding of the disempowered in the practice area. Much work is needed in the use of restraint on vulnerable women who have been the victims of abuse. This practice still occurs and still it traumatises women (Gallop *et al*, 1999). The experience of restraint can undermine all previous gains in personal therapeutic work. Empowering means a rethink on managing restraint so that whatever form it takes, it is very much a final measure.

Myth 3: Healthy caring?

The community, which is strong and empowering, is a community where growth takes place, where all members feel that they have an equal and fair say in how discipline is maintained. The reality of life in general and the institutional community in particular means that such a goal is hard to attain. If both sides of the equation, ie. nurses and patients are not committed to this same goal, then the health of that community is affected. Again, it centres on commonality and a mutual respect for all members. Tones (1998) notes four features of such a community:

1. A feeling of belonging.
2. Shared emotional connection.
3. Influence — a sense that all matter.
4. Integration and fulfilment of needs by group membership.

That community, which is created, has to be a place that is positive and hopeful. That hope is often lost when facilities are poor and when there is a sense of hopelessness in the staff members. Hogg (1999) noted that professional pessimism creates more limited outlooks for the patients and users and hinders their re-integration back into the community. Where the negative nursing voice is loud then the client cannot feel empowered by the healthy community. The voices of those women who have been abused by psychiatry, rather than cared for, are only now being heard. The real tragedy of the situation is that there are many nurses who are caring and involved and would very much like to distance themselves from the past. It is noteworthy how many survivors have commented on this issue and how these nurses are themselves treated by the system.

Realities of empowerment

The WISH perspective

The verb 'empower' is defined as, 'give power to; make able' (*Oxford English Dictionary*, 2002), but this is the antithesis of the current system that discriminates against women. Women account for only 16% of the population in high secure care and 10%–15% in medium secure care. In the latter, a woman may find herself the only woman on a ward of fifteen men. In institutions where women are controlled by disciplined regimes, where issues of custody predominate over sensitive care and treatment, the affective vulnerability, lack of self-identity and sense of powerlessness experienced by women with a borderline personality disorder (BPD) diagnosis is exaggerated. This leads to greater impulsiveness, including self-harming and aggressive behaviour. Statistically, there is a high, disproportionate use of seclusion for women in both medium and high secure care. Hence the labels of difficult, dangerous, manipulative and resultant low status afforded by the staff who work with them. In essence, the women feel threatened, violated and have little or no control over their lives.

This process is exaggerated and of even more concern when we look at the numbers of women diagnosed with BPD, very much a gendered diagnosis. Case Register Data shows that a high proportion of women patients in high secure hospitals are classified as having a personality disorder. Although women make up only 16% of the population in high secure hospitals, on admission, 45% are diagnosed as having a personality disorder compared to 28% of male patients (Case Register Data, 1998). Other research studies indicate that the vast majority of the women in this classification meet the diagnostic criteria for BPD. According to a research study undertaken by Coid (1992), 91% of women within this category meet the diagnostic criteria for BPD.

The process of classification, using the DSM-IV diagnostic criteria, focuses solely on symptoms, open to a wide interpretation, with no reference to any background of severe abuse, which is almost always present. WISH argues unequivocally that the women we represent have been chronically traumatised by their experiences, resulting in enduring personality changes. Herman (1992) suggests that a much more positive model for understanding the difficulties experienced by this group of women, complex post-traumatic stress disorder, should be applied. This model is concerned with causation as well as symptoms. Bloom promotes a trauma based therapeutic model founded on a strong conviction that, although it may require life-long processing, recovery from traumatic experience is possible.

The BPD diagnosis is commonly used by staff to 'describe' a patient, eg. 'Rachel is a borderline'. This practice alone has a dehumanising effect, particularly as the diagnosis carries such negative connotations, creating an even greater distance between patients and staff and deepening the women's sense of disempowerment. The findings of a recent consultation, with fifty-six patients in secure care, indicated that their stories revealed a shared belief that the dream of discharge could best be achieved by toeing the line rather than fully addressing the causes of their distress. With little responsibility or choice over their daily lives and futures, women said, 'we are expected to behave like adults but we get treated like children' (Parry-Crooke, 2000). There are pockets of good practice, but tragically, it is mostly the staff with insight and compassion who leave the secure system as they become as disempowered as the women; they become victims of the parallel process which exists within secure settings.

Within the context of manipulative behaviours staff will also, negatively, refer to these women as having the ability to create 'splits' because they are diagnosed as having a borderline personality disorder. Kernberg (1972, p. 233), in his contributions to the object relations' theory of normal development, postulated four stages in the development of normal internalised object relations:

> *During Stage 4, 'good' and 'bad' self-images coalesce into an integrated self-concept... at the same time 'good' and 'bad' object images also coalesce such that the 'good' and the 'bad' images of mother become integrated into a whole-object conception of mother, which closely approaches the actuality or the reality of mother in the child's interpersonal-perceptual field.*

(Kernberg, 1972, p.233)

Kernberg theorised that the fixation peculiar to the borderline syndrome occurred in the third stage of development, where there still persisted a dissociation of libidinously determined (= good) from aggressively determined (= bad) self and object representations. A consequence of this is the pathological persistence of the primitive defence of splitting.

While staff continue to cast themselves in the role of 'good guy', and by implication patients in the role of 'bad guy', it is hard to see how patients will be empowered to heal this split, least of all be allowed to participate in the process. It is also difficult to understand how a heavy reliance on the medical model will help the women, particularly when opportunities to access appropriate therapies are limited. WISH advocates the development of dedicated, gender sensitive services that reflect the significant essential differences in the women's social and offending profiles (where this applies), their mental distress and complex patterns of behaviour, their care and treatment needs underpinned by the principles of empowerment, respect and dignity.

Reed (1994) suggested that in male-dominated environments, women's needs, including their more personal female needs, are more likely to be overlooked, and they are more likely to suffer sexual harassment and other demeaning behaviour. Reed (1994) went on to propose that to counter this effect there is a need for positive action, and generally to ensure that women receive the care, treatment, accommodation and rehabilitation they need with proper attention to their personal dignity.

Lart *et al* (1998) in a similar vein observed that there is:

A need to facilitate the involvement of women patients as stakeholders in the planning of their care and treatment. This is important not only in relation to empowerment, but also for therapeutic reasons.

Empowerment means actively listening to the women, validating their experiences and facilitating their authentic participation in their care and treatment.

Providing a therapeutic context in which women can begin the process of empowerment essentially means listening to them and making the space and time. A lot of unlearning has to be done by staff before that active listening process can take place. It requires a commitment by staff, as mental health professionals, to suspend their own opinions, experience and knowledge of what women are, what they need, how they should behave and lead their lives. Staff need to give validity to the patient's internal world, rather than putting their own meaning on it. Women need to unlearn, too. Their experience of disempowerment is deep and profound, it is a slow process and it will take time for them to trust. It is the responsibility of the professional to teach and model healthy relationships, within clear, safe and fully explained boundaries. This requires a shift in the power base between patient and professional; it requires staff to work beyond the strict confines of the psychiatric medical model of care.

Students and service users rarely share input to curriculum development

The Department of Health (1994) advocated the involvement of users and carers in the curricula for professional education. Such involvement is now widespread in various centres where professionals are trained. However, it is not yet universal and real involvement is in reality quite limited. In empowering students in this way we are empowering the clients. Where both learn together, both feel able to have therapeutic alliances that will work to initiate change. In situations such as nursing in secure environments, where there are clear boundaries of control, the divide between the novice patient and the expert nurse can be a chasm. If both have had the experience of resolving a care issue in training, neither is so terrified by the other in the care situation.

As educators/workers we need to recognise the importance of sustaining patient power, and explore strategies to reverse the trend when disempowerment is the norm. Wood and Wilson-Barnett (1999) identified the discomfort felt when users were involved in education. Professional socialisation and coping with criticism can lead, not to empowerment, but entrenchment on both sides if not handled appropriately. They note:

> *Listening to users being critical and angry about professional practice can be uncomfortable and lead to professionals becoming defensive. These attitudes are likely to be deep rooted in professional socialisation and may be operating at an unconscious level.*

(Wood and Wilson-Barnett, 1999, p. 259)

Where this can be dealt with sensitively in a learning and safe environment, the confidence to act in this way in situations where change is needed may be easier. Likewise, it seems counter-productive to continue to teach students assertion skills for their future practice if the patient is not taught the same skills. If students can learn assertion skills in dealing with colleagues, they can also apply these skills directly to patient care by acting in a kind of advocacy role with their patients (White, 1998).

The need to understand the effects of earlier abuse on patients with subsequent mental health disturbance should assume a greater prominence in the curricula of all workers in the secure environment. Gallop *et al* (1999) noted the devastation caused by these experiences and what they felt would provide a basis for care. If patients are to be helped then the following criteria are central:

- that they are believed
- that they are heard
- that they are human beings and not just patients with a label and a history.

The authors also note that:

Unfortunately, when nurses perceive themselves as being undervalued or treated with disrespect, there is a risk those feelings will be passed on to the client and expressed in negative nursing behaviours.

(Gallop *et al*, 1999, p. 414)

One of the authors (JR) is at present undertaking research in how survivors describe their self-hatred following abuse, and the narratives expressed to date indicate that students could learn much from hearing some of the stories in the course of their training.

Carers are not cared for

It would seem that if nurses were to empower or attempt to provide an empowering environment which is supportive and caring, they need to feel the same way for themselves. Barker (1998) point out that the 'us and them' mentality is still cogent in care delivery. The authors invite the reader to question how much this has to extend to workers being able to deliver care when they have been or are service users themselves. This is a prime issue since the Clothier Report, following the killing of children by a nurse. The profession has still not dealt fully with the issue of how much a person with past mental distress is capable of being a nurse. What of course is interesting is that we simply do not know who is capable of assault or even murder; there are few indicators that are reliable and even fewer that can be used as a screening process. Barker *et al* (1998) point out that, 'It is axiomatic that no one can assert with any confidence that they will not experience any kind of mental distress in the future'. Maybe nurses need to be enabled to let some users care for them in order to care for others. The vulnerable nurse or other worker is often ignored or made to feel redundant when they are not fully coping with the work or, indeed, their own feelings raised as a result of their work with clients. Indeed, nurses have been criticised for their involvement with so-called difficult patients, including very often those whose diagnosis is of a personality disorder, or who self-harm on a frequent basis (Arnold, 1994; Reece, 1998). If we are to empower our clients we have to support those who work with people with deep-seated distress, rather than be suspicious that maybe they are losing objectivity when there is no real evidence to suggest that this is happening. This, in its turn, means that supervision has also to be non-confrontatory, based not only on skill supervision and development, but also on personal development.

Conclusions

With regard to staff, empowerment has to start at the entry point of training and to be a lived experience for the student. Education must be seen to be empowering, not dehumanising and controlling. Professional skills can still be assessed and attained without the destruction of the student. There also needs to be increased use of service users in all areas of academic study, not just as patients that students are placed to work with.

Is empowerment valid without professional recognition that we have removed power in the first place? When we seek to be empowering why are we undertaking this? Unless we are really prepared to lose power and break down gender discrimination then the approach is simply not valid.

In respect of patients, WISH concludes that if women in secure hospitals are to experience true empowerment they must be involved in their care and treatment and decisions about their lives. It is no longer acceptable for women to be 'done to', particularly women who have endured abuse. Bloom (1998) refers to the need for women and staff to be in a process that forges a 'bridge of compassion'. Care teams need to understand that the patient was and is a person; to understand the sufferings she has endured; and to understand that she developed certain coping skills to survive incredible traumas and remains arrested in her development.

Bloom found that when this understanding was established, staff attitudes towards the patients dramatically changed for the better. The staff no longer felt persecuted or under attack, or experienced resentment and anger towards the patients. This shift in the paradigm of care enabled women, in turn, positively to change their attitudes toward the staff.

Once staff display compassion, slowly the patients can gain some compassion for themselves and for their own suffering. Using this bridge of compassion, patients are more likely to start the process of rebuilding their lives. They start to mature again from the point at which their growth and integrity was arrested.

If empowerment is to exist in the context of secure hospitals, and women are to participate in the process, then perhaps this quote from Moira Potier (1993, p. 26) sums it up:

Women need the space to decide for themselves the impact of their experiences within a framework that provides therapy from a women-centred perspective. There is a passionate need for women to feel genuinely valued, listened to and be entitled to reciprocity of respect and validation.

Key points

⌘ Despite the many advances in society, empowerment for women is far from complete and this is particularly evident in the delivery of health care where diagnostic terminology is often used to perpetuate inequality, and ensure the locus of control remains with the professional.

⌘ Student professionals are socialised into disempowering mindsets, and generally accept that status and the ability to control others is a badge of that profession. They learn the language of 'the expert' and enter a professional hierarchy where the more expert they become, the greater the void between them and the recipient of care.

⌘ A paradox exists between the 'value' placed on a professional by society, and their alienation from their client group. This reinforces a degree of elitism where those who may exercise considerable power and authority are least in touch.

⌘ Recognition that disempowerment exists does not produce empowerment.

⌘ Participation is the key to empowerment for all women receiving care from those in secure hospitals to the GP's surgery.

Reference

Arnold L (1995) *Women and Self-injury: A survey of 76 women*. Bristol Crisis Service for Women (BCSW), Bristol

Barker P *et al* (1998) *Psychiatric Nursing: Ethical strife*. Arnold, London

Bloom S (1998) *Creating Sanctuary — Towards the Evolution of a Sane Society*. Routledge, London

Breeze J, Repper J (1998) Struggling for Control: The care experiences of 'difficult' patients in mental health services. *J Adv Nurs* **28**(6): 1301–11

Candib LM, ed (1994) Reconsidering Power. In: Department of Health (1998) *Working in Partnership: A Collaborative Approach to Care*. DoH, London

Case Register Data (1998) *Antisocial Behaviour: Research Report, 1997–98*. Maudesley Hospital, London

Coid W (1992) DSM III diagnosis in criminal psychopaths: a way forward. *Criminal Behaviour and Mental Health* **2**: 78–79

Cowan WM (1996) *Annual Review of Neuroscience 1996*. Annual Reviews, Toronto

Department of Health (1994) *Our Healthier Nation*. DoH, London

Fraher A, Limpinnian M (1999) User empowerment within mental health nursing. In: Wilkinson G, Miers M, eds. *Power and Nursing Practice*. Macmillan Press, Basingstoke

Fritchie R, Dame (1999) *Secure futures for women: Making a difference*. DoH, London

Gallop R, McCay E, Gula A, Khan P (1999) The experience of hospitalisation and restraint by women who have a history of childhood sexual abuse. *Health Care for Women International* **20**: 401–16

Herman JL (1992) *Trauma and Recovery*. Basic Books, New York

Hogg C (1999) *Patients, Power and Politics from Patients to Citizens*. Sage Publishing, London

Home Office Statistical Bulletin 16/96 *Cautions, Court Proceedings and Sentencing; England and Wales 1995*

Kernberg O (1972) Early ego integration and object relations. *Ann New York Acad Sci* **193**: 233–47

Lart R, Payne S, Beaumont B, Macdonald G, Mistry T (1998) *Women and secure psychiatric services: a literature review*. Report to the NHS Centre for Reviews and Dissemination, University of York

Lloyd A (1995) *Doubly Deviant, Double Damned. Society's Treatment of Violent Women*. Penguin, Harmondsworth

More ES, Milligan M (1994) *The Empathic Practitioner, Empathy Gender and Medicine*. Rutgers University Press, New Brunswick, New Jersey

Mowforth G (1999) Elitism in Nursing. In: Parry-Crooke G (2000) *Good Girls: surviving the secure system*. University of North London, London

Oxford English Dictionary (2002) *Oxford English Dictionary*. Oxford University Press, Oxford

Parry-Crooke G (2000) *Good Girls: Surviving the secure system. A consultation with women in high and medium secure settings*. Women in Secure Hospitals/University of North London, London

Potier MA (1993) Giving evidence. Women's lives in Ashworth maximum security psychiatric hospital. *Feminism Psychology* **3**(3): 335–47

Reece J (1998) Female Survivors of abuse attending A&E with self-injury. *Accid Emerg Nurs* **6**: 133–8

Reed J (1994) *Race, Gender & Equal Opportunities*. vol 6. Review of Health and Social services for mentally disordered offenders and others requiring similar services. HMSO , London

Stafford P (1999) *Defining Gender Issues... redefining women's services* (1). WISH, London

Tones K (1998) Empowerment for Health: The challenge. In: Kendall S, ed (1998) *Health and Empowerment: Research and Practice*. Arnold, London

White H (1998) Improving advocacy and partnerships: reflection on a critical incident. *Paediatr Nurs* **10**(9): 14–16

Wilkinson G, Miers M (1999) *Power and Nursing Practice*. Macmillan, Basingstoke

Wood J, Wilson-Barnett J (1999) The Influence of user involvement on the learning of mental health nursing students. *Nurs Times Res* **4**(4): 257–70

Wollstonecraft M (1792) *A Vindication of the Rights of Women*. (1995). Pheonix, London

8

Empowerment and ethnicity

Mel Chevannes

This chapter provides a brief review of the literature on patient empowerment. Discussion about empowerment in contemporary health care has paid little attention to the ethnicity of patients in spite of the assumed benefits for individuals (Gibson, 1991; National Health Service Management Executive [NHS ME], 1993). The chapter begins by exploring the early origins of the use of the concept of empowerment and moves to contextualise the discussion by examining its meanings in health care by focusing on patients. Crucial to an examination of empowerment of minority ethnic patients is the inclusion and evaluation of accounts of some of these individuals when they turn to the health service for care and treatment. In keeping with the spirit, if not the experience of patient empowerment, four patients' views are incorporated to reflect recent official advocacy for patient involvement (DoH, 1999).

Early origins

For over twenty years, the concept of empowerment has been present in discussion. Some writers claim that the idea of empowerment is associated with the pre-1970s community movement and feminism. This movement emphasised citizenship, collective responsibility and community (Anderson, 1996; WHO, 1998). Others argue that the idea has its origins in radical socialist thought, as in critical social theory, where the interests of individuals, in contrast to those of the state, are necessary to enable people to achieve their full potential (Habermas, 1972). In more recent times, the idea of empowerment has become part of the accepted discourse on individualism, although in the absence of ethnicity.

Context of health care

Empowerment of patients in contemporary health care has received much attention and support, possibly on the assumption that it is a good thing, leads to health improvement, and to patients being healthier. A review of the literature on patient empowerment emphasises these generalised outcomes, but as Elliott and Turrell (1996, p. 46) caution, it is necessary 'to define what we mean by this term (empowerment) and ensure that our definition is meaningful in the clinical area'. This plea emphasises the capacity of implementing empowerment in ways that patients can see and understand.

Three broad meanings of patient empowerment emerge from the review of the relevant literature:

- a social process of enhancement
- a transfer of power
- a package of rights.

Empowerment as a social process leading to enhancement of patients

Gibson (1991, p. 359) describes empowerment as a social process of enhancement for patients in the following way:

> *A social process of recognising, promoting and enhancing peoples' abilities to meet their own needs, solve their own problems and mobilise the necessary resources in order to feel in control of their lives.*

In the context of nursing, the above definition emphasises that nurses should actively support patients, providing clear information about their particular health status and clinical care, so that individuals can participate in decisions being made. Equally important is that such a process will enable patients to take the lead in discussions about their assessment and care with nurses and other health professionals. In practice, there are likely to be different clinical situations where patients may be supported to put their points of view and others where the patients' empowerment is at the level of being fully informed about assessment, care and the treatment to be provided. Nurses and other health professionals need to recognise empowerment when patients 'do' things as well as 'know' about the care. But as Elliott and Turrell (1996, p. 227) make clear, patients being involved in decisions about their care and whether 'that involvement is recognised as empowering or not, is far from self-evident'.

The assumed benefits of empowerment for patients who meet their own needs (health and social care), problem-solve, and achieve the resources necessary to exercise control over their lives imply that 'empowerment' is there to be taken by patients. The assumed benefits also suggest that the concept of empowerment is capable of being applied in different acute and primary care situations in which patients find themselves.

The above definition by Gibson (1991) also assumes that all patients are willing to exercise choice to enter the process of enhancement and to exit at any stage. There can be no guarantee that all patients, ethnic minority and ethnic majority, will recognise the benefits of empowerment as prescribed, or that nurses and other health professionals will positively promote the process all, or even some of the time, irrespective of the implication of their role in the care. This point follows into the second meaning of 'empowerment'.

Empowerment as a transfer of power

Empowerment defined as a transfer of power implies that there is a quantifiable sum that is capable of being shared among the participants involved in a process of care. The NHS ME (1993) describes empowerment as a shift in the amount of power from nurses and other health professionals, to people who use health services. Gibson (1991) also argues that nurses need to give up their power and assist patients to gain control. Both meanings suggest that power is a constant sum, and if one person gains the other loses. Furthermore, that patients are powerless or have less power throughout a consultation or episode of care compared with the nurse or health professional involved. It is important to note that the literature highlights the transfer of power as pivotal to achieving patient empowerment, yet the debate is often imprecise about the role of patients in the care team. These empowered patients are variously described, as essential advisors (Price, 1986), genuine participants (Ashworth *et al*, 1992), collaborators (Jewell, 1994), and equal partners (Gibson, 1991). This equivocation over the role of the empowered patient, indicates a degree of vagueness and/or generalisation about a state/status and remains inconclusive. Genuine participants can be effective in action which can be disputed, while equal partners in the process of care can be more easily measured and agreed.

A package of rights

A third meaning of empowerment in health care is the idea of defining rights for patients and other individuals. The National Health Service Management Executive (NHS ME, 1993) describes this view and advocates six rights of equal value to be provided in all care settings with patients. The six rights include:

❖ Equal access to health services for all. Patients' access to services needs to take account of peoples' social class, ethnicity, age, gender, economic circumstances, physical and mental capacity in deciding on the location, design, and delivery of health care to reduce inequalities at local level.

❖ Fair treatment and redress in dealing with complaints by patients and/or their advocates. Here, information about complaint procedures needs to be publicly available, operate in a simple and straightforward way to achieve speedy and fair resolutions.

❖ Patients should be given the choice to be represented at any stage in an episode of care. Patients' choice should be respected and supported by all health professionals.

❖ Consent of patients should be sought before they participate in audit and development of services. The issue of patients' consent is a fundamental principle which healthcare professionals are required to obtain and not assume.

❖ Patients or clients should be respected for exercising their autonomy in decisions that are being made about their care and/or treatment.

❖ Maximum information should be provided about care given and services that are available.

The six rights outlined above are offered as a package to patients and, by implication, included in their care plan. The rights are very much the policy makers' expectations of the care provided by the National Health Service. The challenge for nurses and healthcare professionals is how to translate the six rights into tangible benefits that patients can see and experience. For example, providing maximum health information to patients about care on offer and services available, does not necessarily lead to understanding by patients. Having a shared language (verbal and written) between patients, nurses and other health professionals is vital to receiving information and understanding by all individuals involved in the interaction.

In a discussion about empowering older people through communication, Le May (1998) argues that a multifaceted approach should be adopted to reflect their diversity, based on health needs and their knowledge of specific disease from which they may be at risk. From an Age Concern (1996) commissioned national survey of 1033 older women, 24% believed that they were at high risk of developing breast cancer, or knew that they had a right to request breast screening. On the basis of this finding, Age Concern concluded that health information about breast cancer failed to reach women aged sixty-five years and over, a group which is most at risk of developing the disease. Clearly, there is a long way to go before the health services can claim that they have provided sufficient information to those who are at risk of developing a particular disease. The idea of patients being empowered by receiving maximum information challenges those responsible for communicating to ensure that the language is appropriate, terms are explained in a straightforward manner, and different approaches to communication are utilised.

The issue of communicating information as a step towards patient empowerment is also crucial for some minority ethnic patients who do not speak or understand the language used by the nurse. Reliable and appropriate interpreters can usefully bridge the communication gap and improve the understanding of both patients and staff of the patients' condition.

The three broad meanings of empowerment in health care and a review of the literature more generally, omit any explicit reference to ethnicity, or more specifically to patients from minority ethnic groups (Anderson, 1996; Gibson, 1991; Rapport, 1984; Elliott and Turrell, 1996; NHS ME, 1993). National health policy (DoH, 1997, p. 2000) emphasises the need to consider patients, users, and carers in their social context and to do so more explicitly in decisions which affect their care. This position can be seen as a starting point towards working with patients, within safe but often different practices, for their health improvement. Crucial to what McDougall (1997) refers to as a 'fundamental way of thinking and working', is a particular way of working. It is argued that nurses and health professionals need to think of patients as partners in the care process. This approach is necessary to develop a culture of equality between all the partners (more popularly described as partnership working).

In an attempt to contextualise the discussion about the meanings of empowerment in health care, use is made of patients' experience by the case study method. The users are drawn from black and other minority ethnic groups and from the white majority ethnic group.

Three questions are used to structure the accounts of five users of the National Health Service:

- are patients, irrespective of their ethnicity group, empowered in the context of health care?
- what does empowerment mean for them?
- who decides when they are empowered and how?

To proceed to gain a response to the questions from the point of view of the individuals, five scenarios are developed below. An attempt will be made to relate as far as possible the evaluation of the scenarios to the three broad meanings of empowerment examined earlier in the chapter.

Scenario 1

A fifty-eight-year-old Indian woman, a housewife, was referred to a local acute hospital by her general practitioner because of generalised pain across her abdomen. As she was being assessed in a medical assessment unit of the acute hospital NHS trust, she told the nurse, in English, that she had, and pointed as she said this, pain all over her stomach. The pain started a day ago. She also said that she had not eaten any meals for a few days, thought that something was seriously wrong, and that she was very anxious. The nurse nodded her head and said, 'I understand'.

The woman's history was recorded by the nurse who also carried out some further assessment, including blood pressure, temperature and pulse reading. The assessment of all three were within normal limits and the woman was informed. The nurse did not provide any explanation about the questions she asked of the woman. Throughout the whole process of taking the woman's history, the nurse was more determined to pursue with questioning the woman rather than offering information about the symptoms she described.

The doctor also carried out an assessment of the patient. When she touched her abdomen (with warm hands) the patient complained of pain. With her face twisted in agony, she said in a gasp, 'I know something is wrong with my stomach'. The doctor responded and said 'we will find out'. She did not provide any indication of the course of action she planned to take or when anything would happen.

Was this older Indian woman patient empowered in the above interaction with the nurse and the doctor in the medical assessment unit? Was her ability to describe when the pain started, her inability to eat, and symptoms about the pain all in her stomach, a dimension of empowerment? The patient communicated in the language that the nurse and doctor understood. The patient used the word 'stomach' and pointed to the area of her body to which she referred.

The patient's verbal and non-verbal communication about the pain enabled the nurse and doctor to carry out a thorough assessment. The patient, nurse and doctor contributed different kinds of knowledge and skills to the assessment process, without any obvious loss of power from the two professionals. However, the woman was given very little information about what constituted 'normal' blood pressure, temperature and pulse readings. She was not provided with any information about the purpose of the questions, the care she could expect or any choice she had in the process.

In the above scenario, patient empowerment may be seen as her ability to describe symptoms of pain. The key issues for empowerment include:

❖ The patient is able to describe the symptoms in a language she is confident to use.

❖ Clear communication, which is understood by patient, nurse and doctor.

❖ Communication by the patient to describe symptoms of pain she experienced, her inability to eat meals, when the pain started, her response when the doctor touched her abdomen, and an expression of pain by facial expression.

❖ Nurse and doctor hear the patient's story but without sharing information about what they intend to do or providing her with choice about care.

❖ The patient requirement for professional help with diagnosis, care and treatment are not explained.

Scenario 2

Mrs C is a seventy-eight-year old Black Caribbean woman who had diabetes diagnosed three years after she retired from work as a seamstress. Her diabetes was controlled by oral medication, one metformin tablet, 850 milligram, three times per day, and a moderate intake of Caribbean food. Initially, she used Labstix (a reagent strip test dipped in fresh urine to test for pH, protein, glucose, ketones and blood) to test her urine for sugar on a daily basis. This test was no longer routinely necessary. She did, however, decide to use this test when she felt it was needed.

She recalled one consultation with the practice nurse when she attended for a check up about the diabetes. She remarked that the nurse said that if the diabetes was in the urine, it was also in the blood. She added that the nurse told her that if the diabetes was not controlled by the tablets she would have to get the injection, but quickly retorted, 'she did not threaten me though, she was being honest'. Although Mrs C was being provided with information about the prescribed tablets to control her diabetes and the possibility that she could receive the medication by injection, the information was not offered as a choice of treatment.

On another occasion when she had finished the metformin tablets as prescribed, she visited the practice for a repeat prescription. Prior to the visit, she had made repeated phone calls to the practice as well as left a stamped addressed envelope for the prescription to be signed by the GP and posted to her home. One month passed and no prescription had arrived. She said:

> *I was feeling sick without the tablet, my head was heavy and I felt giddy. When I eventually got an appointment to see my GP, the practice nurse was cross saying that I needed the tablets and should not have gone without them. When she was asked who the nurse was cross with, she replied 'that they [the practice] did not call me for the prescription'.*

Mrs C viewed nurses and doctors as clever and relied heavily on their comments. After fifteen years of consultation with her general practitioner, practice nurse, hospital consultants and nurses, she was confident to recall the commentary and advice of these professionals with little or no questioning. When she was questioned about her diabetes by family members, she occasionally expressed irritation that 'maybe they [the doctors and nurses] don't know what they do'. For example, when, as an outpatient, she was examined by a hospital doctor to assess the severity of arthritis which was affecting her hips and knees, the doctor (reported) said that she had 'bruising of the bones' and nothing could be done because of the diabetes. The doctor did not provide any information about what could be done.

She talked confidently about having a cataract in both eyes which was caused by diabetes but did not have a discussion with the doctor about the likelihood of having either of the cataracts removed. During one of her hospital consultations she was told that she would have an operation to remove the cataract from one eye. Mrs C was not given a choice but accepted what she was told by the doctor, as her sight would improve. She has had a successful operation on one eye. No information has been provided about whether she would have the other cataract removed or if there is a choice of treatment.

Her understanding of diabetes, the effects on her vision and her management of oral medication have been gained from consultations with professionals over a fifteen-year period. She managed her diet by having Caribbean meals and coped with her social and religious life.

Is Mrs C an empowered patient during the consultations outlined above or in the way that she uses the knowledge gained about diabetes to manage her life?

Scenario 3

Mr E is a seventy-eight-year-old Black Caribbean man who had diabetes diagnosed ten years after retirement from paid work as a car worker in the paint department. His diabetes was controlled broadly with oral medication.

Mr E has limited understanding of scientific and technical knowledge about diabetes and most other medical matters. He followed his medication regimen, by taking one glibenclamide tablet, 5 milligram daily. Mr E managed his diabetes with Caribbean foods and oral medication. He decided about his meals, kind and quantity (excluding sugar and sweets) in terms of what he liked and has used over many years. His test of foods which complement the diabetes was based on the stability of sugar in the urine, maintenance of his body weight, and his general feeling of well-being.

He talked about his diabetes in his own words with his added interpretations. He was happy to relate how he managed the diabetes in the following way:

I know how I feel — I'm not giddy or tired.
I feel good when I do the shopping with my wife.
I eat the Caribbean foods I like but I also take the tablet everyday.
I do not rely very much on doctors because they don't explain what they do or give you much information.
They [the doctors and the nurses too] treat you as if you don't matter.
They behave as if you are there for them rather than the other way round.

The above comments provided by Mr E indicate that he is trying to manage his diabetes with Caribbean foods and intake of tablets. He believes that he was given little information to help him understand diabetes. He also believes that his sense of well-being is lowered in his consultation with doctors and nurses. Is Mr E empowered in the description provided?

Scenario 4

Mr R is a sixteen-year-old young man of English and black Caribbean heritage. He took a break from revising for general certificates in secondary education in eleven subjects to play football. While he was playing football he felt his left knee weakened. He fell to the ground, as he had no support in his left knee. When he hopped home, a few metres from where he was playing football, his father took him to the local accident and emergency department. After registration in the department and having to wait four hours before being assessed by a doctor, his father took him back home.

Within the four hours, Mr R accompanied by his father and mother returned to the accident and emergency department. Mr R and his mother were shown in a cubicle by a nurse. Shortly afterwards, a doctor came into the cubicle and without looking at his mother or smiling at him, asked Mr R what had happened to his knee. He responded about the incident when he was playing football earlier in the evening. After an assessment of the left knee, the doctor told him that it was bruised and that a nurse would come to see him. The mother asked the doctor what he meant. He turned as though he was surprised and looked at her for the first time and said, 'he has injured his knee and the nurse will explain'.

The nurse came in shortly afterwards, smiled at Mr R and told him that she would put a support over his knee. She left and returned a few minutes later and said that she could not find a tubigrip applicator. The mother offered to put the support on her son's left knee if she would cut the required length. This action was agreed. After the support was put on, the nurse gave Mr R a leaflet about exercises and the application of an ice pack to the knee. She also told him that he should remove the support before he goes to bed.

As Mr R and his parents left the accident and emergency department, Mr R volunteered the information below:

The nurse was nice. She smiled when she spoke with me. I felt good and felt she noticed me as someone with an injury who needed help. The doctor was grumpy. He behaved as if he didn't want to be there, I was a nuisance. He neither looked at me nor smiled.

Scenario 5

Miss F is an eighty-seven-year-old English lady, an ex-art teacher from a secondary school. She lives with her dog. She has occasional visits by friends who live great distances away and a nephew and his wife who live five miles away, but both are in full-time work and work takes them some thirty-six and fifty-five miles respectively, away from their home. These friends and relatives take her out for drives to the outskirts of the town in which she lives, shopping, and visiting relatives. Socially she feels isolated and gets frustrated at having to rely on others to take her out of the bungalow. Her mental health is good but she does not wish to continue to plan the maintenance on the property, as she says 'it has become too much for me, I don't want to continue with this'.

Miss F suffers with glaucoma in both eyes and has had a cataract operation recently to one eye. She has swollen legs but no accompanying medical diagnosis has been made. Her mobility around the bungalow is limited with a walking stick, and she gets breathless. She has difficulty in getting up from a hard tip-up chair. She manages to cook her meals by sitting on a perching stool provided by the Aids for Daily Living Centre which is managed by the local social services department, and is helped to have showers at the bungalow by a bath seat which she places across the bath. She also uses a commode during the nights because of her mobility and fear of having a fall. A raised seat is also permanently situated over the lavatory to help her to get back to standing position with some effort.

Socially, she is keen to continue to sketch and paint, although she is unable to throw pots and practice sculpting at the local adult education centre she visited previously by using the Ring and Ride service. The restricted mobility has reduced the frequency of her attendance to the centre and she greatly regrets losing her artistic skills. She recounts to me:

I enjoy my art, it keeps my brain going, and I want to continue to have a purpose for living. Without my art, my purpose for living with dignity and respect will be gone. I am fed up.

Miss F is ruggedly independent and has little intention, if she can avoid it, of relying on others — friends, relatives or the local social services department — for assistance, except on her terms. However, she has been angry and frustrated since early in the year. She was informed by a friend about a sheltered housing accommodation in the town where she lives. The brochure positively showed that the range of accommodation is designed to meet the different needs of older people. Pictures of an art studio, nursery shop, space, older people with their pets generated great enthusiasm for Miss F. She asked her nephew to take her to visit the sheltered housing.

She duly submitted two different applications as she was instructed to do, and received a response from the applications to the local housing department three months later that she was not allocated any points on medical, social or accommodation criteria. Having no response from the second application about the sheltered housing accommodation by the end of six months, she asked her nephew's wife for help. Acting as an advocate for Miss F, a letter was sent to the director of the social services setting out broadly the views of Miss F. Stress was put on Miss F's need to have company with other people, to remain active while she could still walk, to be relieved of the responsibility of housework and repairs to the bungalow, and, above all, to retain her independence.

Miss F has since been visited at her bungalow by a social worker with her nephew's wife in attendance by invitation.

The social worker was totally focused on the completion of numerous pages of a document, asking Miss F questions about her physical and mental health. Her nephew's wife was almost totally ignored. The social worker sought hard to get a description of a medical diagnosis while Miss F stressed how she was keen to manage her affairs, maintain her independence and to get out of the bungalow. After Miss F's insistence by repetition of these issues, the social worker changed her style of questioning and informed her about getting a call link to be placed around her neck. Miss F said that a call link would not have helped her recently when she fell in her garden at the back of the bungalow. There was some disagreement between the social worker and Miss F about whether the call link would have been effective for that purpose. Miss F informed the social worker that she would need to be in the vicinity of the telephone for the call link to work.

The social worker also informed her about other facilities such as visiting a day centre, accessing private house cleaning agencies and the name of another sheltered housing. The social worker had completed the document at this stage.

After the interview, Miss F said:

> *That was a waste of time. I am being ignored because I am not ill. I want to keep my independence but I am isolated, need to meet people, and to continue with my art. I don't want anything to do with the Council. I really fear having a fall and becoming ill as others will take over my life.*

What are your views on Miss F's wish to retain control of her life and of her contact with health professionals? Was she empowered and, if so, in what sense, when she responded to the brochure in which a sheltered housing was advertised? Was she empowered during the discussion with the social worker? It was clear that she struggled to get an effective response to her needs; she has identified her fear of having a fall, becoming ill as a result and others making decisions about her future.

Discussion of empowerment in the context of patients' views

The scenarios above describe the experience of five patients: two of whom received assessment and treatment at acute hospitals, two of whom received care on a long-term basis provided by general practice and hospital, and one who lived on her own in a bungalow and was in need of support. Three of the patients were older women; one is Indian, one black Caribbean and one English (white). The other two were men; one black Caribbean and the other mixed race.

The descriptions of the consultations were obtained by talking with the five patients following their experiences. It is important to note that none of the patients used the word 'empowerment' in conversation, yet the literature on patient empowerment and the use of the word by healthcare professionals and others remains popular. The selected review of the literature examined in this chapter identifies three broad meanings of patient empowerment: as a social process of enhancement (Gibson, 1991); a transfer of power from professionals to patients (Price, 1986; Gibson, 1991; Ashworth *et al*, 1992; NHS ME, 1993; Jewell, 1994); and as a package of rights (NHS ME, 1993).

In the five scenarios, the patients were managing their lives as best they could against the presence of a disease (diabetes), the context of an acute illness/injury, and in dealing with the effects of the ageing process. They tried to be in control during their consultations and their experiences. The Indian woman in the medical assessment unit, for example, displayed evidence of control over her life, despite being in the midst of excruciating pain. None of the scenarios provides evidence of the transfer of power from professionals to patients or the reality of a right to determine one's own health treatment. In fact, Miss F demonstrated frustration, anger, and a real struggle to retain control within the context of decline in health and growing frailty caused by the ageing process. Rather than patient empowerment being realised as a process of enhancement (Gibson, 1991), Miss F was forced to accept that her existing inadequate arrangements might have to continue and to feel that all her efforts to control her life amounted to nothing.

Elliott and Turrell (1996) have argued that patient empowerment is far from self-evident in practice. Also, that the reality of patient empowerment should be clearly understood by them and seen to be working in health care. The evidence of patient empowerment or lack of it, as in the five scenarios, show that the five individuals, irrespective of age, gender, ethnicity and previous occupation, have a common experience. None of the descriptions convey patient empowerment.

The five scenarios suggest that, the very idea of empowering patients should be challenged as patients try against the odds to exercise their knowledge and skills in their consultations with nurses and other health professionals. They do so without waiting for an invitation or encouragement to put forward their views about their health. More pointedly, they are manipulated away from their expression of need. Patients, differentiated by age, gender, ethnicity and previous occupation have realistic perceptions about health, specific and general. Their perceptions involve making priorities in their lives at times of acute illness or in the face of a long-term condition, or in managing the effects of the ageing process. They also evaluate the usefulness of prescribed medication and care and assess the benefits. They continue to manage their lives within the context of families, on their own or other social groups. It is in this sense that it is more realistic to think of empowering patients, not from the premise of their being powerless, but as individuals with views and under-standing about their illnesses and social life which deserve to be heard by nurses and other health professionals. By listening to patients, including young people, and understanding their experiences and emotions, it is possible to construct ways of working and writing care plans which match patients' priorities and needs.

Conclusion

This chapter has attempted to do two things. Firstly, to consider the origins of empowerment both conceptually and practically and, secondly, to test the reality of empowerment through genuine patient experience.

The discussion relating the application of empowerment to the context of health care, generated three broad meanings of patient empowerment; social process of enhancement, the transfer of power from professionals to patients and a package of rights. These, however, do not constitute a conclusive representation of patient empowerment, and the literature seems to be preoccupied with the concept rather than the practical application.

The description of five real experiences conveys a rather disappointing picture of a lack of empowerment at best and active disempowerment at worst. In particular, scenario number five, highlighted a sense of loss and failure for a woman whose lack of medical diagnosis seemed to indicate that she had no needs. A worrying pattern emerges of patients having to struggle to maintain dignity in consultation with healthcare professionals, and the professionals seeming indifference to the genuine needs of their client group.

Key points

⌘ Empowerment may not always be a good thing, particularly if it is imposed.

⌘ A package of rights, transfer of power or social process of enhancement are fundamental to the concept of empowerment.

⌘ Empowered patients are given information about the purpose, expectations and choices that are available to them. Professionals may encounter difficulties in communicating these elements, because of language or cultural barriers. Professionals should still try and possibly call on outside services that can relate the ideas more effectively.

⌘ Simple, genuine communication is valued by patients; honesty and information together with friendly and appropriate non-verbal communication improve patient satisfaction.

⌘ The five scenarios provide examples where experience fails to convey empowerment despite age, gender, ethnicity or previous occupation.

References

Age Concern (1996) *Not at my age! Why the present breast screening system is failing women aged 65 or over*. Age Concern, London

Anderson J (1996) Empowering patients: issues and strategies. *Soc Sci Med* **43**(5): 697–705

Ashworth PD, Longmate MA, Morrison P (1992) Patient participation: its meaning and significance in the context of caring. *J Adv Nurs* **17**: 1430–9

Clark P (1996) Communication between provider and patient: values, biography and empowerment in clinical practice. *Ageing and Society* **16**: 747–74

Department of Health (1997) *The new NHS — modern, dependable*. Cm 3807. DoH, London

Department of Health (1999) *Patient and public involvement in the new NHS*. DoH, London

Department of Health (2000) *The NHS Plan. A plan for investment. A plan for reform*. DoH, London

Elliott MA, Turrell AR (1996) Dilemmas for the empowering nurse. *J Nurs Management* **4**: 273–9

Gibson C (1991) A concept analysis of empowerment. *J Adv Nurs* **16**(3): 354–61

Habermas J (1972) *Knowledge and Human Interest*. Translated by Shapiro JJ. Heinemann, London

Jewell SE (1994) Patient participation: what does it mean to nurses? *J Adv Nurs* **19**: 433–8

Le May A (1998) Empowering older people through communication. In: Kendall S, ed. *Health and Empowerment*. Arnold, London

McDougall T (1997) Patient empowerment: fact or fiction? *Ment Health Nurs* **17**: 4–5

National Health Service Management Executive (1993) *Patient Empowerment*. NHS ME, Leeds

Price R (1986) Giving the patient control. *Nurs Times* **82**(20): 28–30

Rapport J (1984) Studies in Empowerment: introduction to the issue. *Prevent Inhuman Services* **3**: 1–7

Roter D, Hall J (1992) *Doctors talking with Patients: Patients talking with Doctors*. Auburn House, Westport

World Health Organization (1978) *Alma Ata 1978: Primary Health Care*. WHO, Geneva

9

Age and isms: older people and power

Sally Rudge

Population growth is one of the most significant global problems currently faced by humanity. The demographic trend since industrialisation has produced a change in the equilibrium between young and old people. With the decline in the birth rate and an increase in longevity, older people now make up a large proportion of the population in all industrialised countries. Statistics show that in 1800 the average age of the population was approximately sixteen years. Today, it has reached over thirty-five years.

With the increase in numbers, there comes a reduction in the importance and status within the community given to older people by the rest of the population, so much so that they are often perceived in a negative manner compared to their previous prestigious and powerful positions of earlier years (Riley, 1987). This negative and stereotypic perception of ageing and older individuals is readily apparent in such areas as language, media, and humour. For example, such commonly used phrases as 'over the hill' and 'don't be an old fuddy-duddy' denote old age as a period of impotency and incompetence (Nuessel, 1982).

Butler coined the term ageism in 1969. He likened it to other forms of bigotry such as racism and sexism, defining it as a process of systematic stereotyping and discrimination against people because they are old. More recently the definition has been broadened by Palmore (1990) to incorporate any prejudice or discrimination against or in favour of an age group.

Ageism is not a universal, cross-cultural phenomenon. There appears to be a great variation as to the treatment that older adults receive, ranging from extreme reverence and respect to abandonment and deprivation.

The more modernised the society is, the more likely they are to be ageist and maintain negative attitudes about the aged. Women's status and power does increase in many cultures following menopause (Brown, 1985). Okada (1962, cited in Gutmann, 1985), states that the old widow has great power in the Japanese family. Post-menopausal women in these traditional societies usually experience greater sexual freedom, the right to participate in ritual, the right to participate in the political realm of the society, and a decrease in the amount of work required in the home. With regard to work, the older woman is expected to be leisured.

Where ageism exists, Palmore (1990, pp. 151–152) lists seven basic characteristics of stereotyping that form its basis:

* ❖ The stereotype gives a highly exaggerated picture of the importance of a few characteristics.
* ❖ Some stereotypes are invented with no basis in fact, and are made to seem reasonable by association with other tendencies that have a kernel of truth.
* ❖ In a negative stereotype, favourable characteristics are either omitted entirely or insufficiently stressed.
* ❖ The stereotype fails to show how the majority share the same tendencies or have other desirable characteristics.
* ❖ Stereotypes fail to give any attention to the cause of the tendencies of the minority group — particularly to the role of the majority itself and its stereotypes, in creating the very characteristics being condemned.
* ❖ Stereotypes leave little room for change; there is a lag in keeping up with the tendencies that actually typify many members of the group.
* ❖ Stereotypes leave little room for individual variation, which is particularly wide among elders.

Ageism is different from other 'isms', such as sexism and racism, for two main reasons. Firstly, age classification is not static. An individual's age classification changes as one progresses through the life cycle. Other classifications, such as race and gender, remain constant throughout an individual's life. Secondly, no one is exempt from achieving the status of old age unless they die prematurely at an early age.

Ageism is perpetuated by many negative stereotypes and myths concerning the older adult. For example, Atchley (1985) found that a common belief among the general population was that the majority of over sixty-fives lived in hospital or homes, and the large proportion of them were also senile. The research findings were significantly different. Only 5% of the over sixty-fives lived in accommodation other than their own, and just 7% of the sixty-five to seventy-nine-year-olds had any senility.

Traxler (1980) proposes that four factors have contributed to the negative image of ageing. The first is the fear of death in Western society. It is not only the elderly as individuals that are subject to ageism in our society, but the concept of ageing which is seen as a negative process of decay, and decline in a person's physical and mental state. Taken to its natural end, the ageing process ends in the death of the individual. Western civilisation conceptualises death as outside of the human life cycle (Butler and Lewis, 1977). Death is not seen as a natural and inevitable part of living. This is in contrast to Eastern philosophy where life and death are all part of a continuous cycle. Consequently, for the majority of those with Western society beliefs, death is feared. This personal fear for many people is projected as a negative opinion towards elderly people in general, which is reflected in their behaviour and language. Our society allows this to continue by not addressing this real fear.

The second factor is the general emphasis on the youth culture. For example, throughout the popular media, there is an over-whelming focus on youth, physical beauty, and sexuality. Older adults are primarily ignored or portrayed negatively (Northcott, 1975). The emphasis on youth not only affects how older individuals are perceived but also how older individuals perceive themselves. Persons who are dependent on physical appearance and youth for their identity are likely to experience loss of self-esteem with age (Block *et al*, 1981).

Productivity in terms of economic potential is the third factor contributing to ageism. Both ends of the life cycle are viewed as unproductive: children and the aged. Butler (1969) proposed that middle-aged individuals perceive themselves as carrying the burdens imposed by both groups. Children, however, are viewed as having future economic potential and are a worthwhile investment. Economically, older adults are perceived as a financial liability. Upon retirement, the older adult is no longer viewed as economically productive in Western society and thus devalued.

The final factor contributing to ageism is the published results from early studies on old age. Poorly controlled gerontological studies have reinforced the negative image of the older adult. When ageing was originally studied, researchers went to long-term care institutions where the aged were easy to find. However, as only 5% of the older population are being cared for away from their home, their findings were invalid for the large majority of older people.

Ageist attitudes are also perpetuated across the media and Western culture. A negative image of old age is portrayed in advertisements, TV programmes, birthday cards and everyday language. Ageist comments are so common within language that people may not realise that they have made one. Phrases such as, 'old hag', 'old maid', 'old fogey' and 'dirty old man' are used freely in our society, and the speaker is not viewed as having said something sociably unacceptable as they would have been had they said something racist or sexist.

Differences between young and old adults' approaches to life may be a cause of frustration, which in turn leads to ageism. As one reaches retirement there is much more free time to manage. People may use this time to reminisce and reflect on the passed times, continually looking back at the 'good old days'. Although reminiscence and reflection are seen as a healthy necessity to achieve successful ageing, too much can be detrimental, and younger adults may find such discussions a waste of time as their priorities are of the here and now and the future, planning and providing for their lives and the lives of their offspring.

It is generally accepted that the pace of life today is faster than in previous years, partly due to the advances in technology. There is a growing difference between the time individuals have got to complete tasks each day. The elderly seeming to have plenty of time, consequently take time, while the young working adult is pressured from work and the media to perform increasingly well in work, leisure and home-life. This may cause great frustration and resentment, again leading to ageism.

Ageing bias is culturally transmitted from adults to their children. The same misconceptions and beliefs about the elderly and the ageing process can be seen replicated between both ages (Pratt, 1981; Seefeldt, 1989).

Old people are often too timid or polite to challenge actively discrimination on an individual basis and, in addition, institutions perpetuate ageism. Businesses frequently reinforce ageist stereotypes by not appointing or promoting older workers. They prefer instead to appoint 'young blood' or graduates into positions in preference to the older 'unwilling to change with the times', or 'unable to grasp new concepts' person.

Within the health service there is a major recruitment drive, led by the Government, to train more people to be nurses as they have predicted a need for nursing staff in the future to care for the ageing population.

As there is no legal retirement age for nurses, and there are many nurses not wanting to retire at sixty-five years old, studies should find this older age group of nurses still in practice, thus alleviating the staffing crisis. Recent findings show that ageist practices are ending careers, before the individuals feel ready for retirement (Coombes, 1999a).

Recent Department of Health figures indicate that there are only ninety qualified nurses aged over sixty-five years working for the National Health Service. An explanation for this sharp reduction in staff numbers could be attributed to the power management staff have to use other policies, such as the Health and Safety at Work Act, in order to create an illusion of a retirement age, which can be used against those individuals who want to continue to practice. To address this issue, the Government has produced a code of practice, *The Diversity in Employment Code of Practice* (NHS Executive, 1999). This is aimed at all trusts and primary care groups, encouraging them to eliminate the use of age as an employment criterion, and to allow retirement to be a phased process. There is no supporting legal requirement to adhere to this code of practice. Consequently, staff who are subject to ageist practices will not be able to use this document in employment tribunals, as it is not statutory. While seemingly supporting and working towards anti-ageist practices, the Government are not giving any additional power to the older person, the power base remaining with the health service.

In recent years, there have been organisations that acknowledge the skills and experience of the older worker as opposed to the younger employee who has not had the time or the opportunity to develop their skills to such an extent. Also, an older person is less likely to move jobs, and this steady, settled behaviour can have a beneficial influence on the work culture, and reduces the problems related to recruitment and selection. As yet, the National Health Service is not one such organisation. Private nursing homes appear less ageist in their employment opportunities, with one home found to be employing a seventy-seven-year-old nurse (Coombes, 1999b).

As the population is ageing, the majority will now experience old age rather than the minority of earlier years. Stokes (1995) predicts that most elderly people living in our society will not have a happy and fulfilling old age, and should expect poor health, neglect by their children and family, and abandonment by their community. They are likely to be ignored and forced to lead a solitary life, living their last years in an institution of some kind, ie. they will be subject to ageism.

Socially, the elderly are ignored as they are seen to be 'boring' or senile, while family members may find them hard work and sickly, a burden. Ill health and disability is a common prejudice against the older person. American studies have shown that around half of the under sixty-fives think that their elders suffer very serious problems with their health (Harris, 1981, cited in Palmore, 1990). They are more prone to accidents, have poor coordination, sleep for greater periods of time and are less immune to infection.

Further studies have contradicted these beliefs. Soldo and Manton (1983) calculated that 81% of people aged over sixty-five years live in their own accommodation without their experiencing significant limitations to their activities of daily living skills. Both British and American studies indicate that older people are healthier than perceived. There are fewer acute illnesses, accidents and injuries compared to the younger cohort (Palmore, 1986). There are lower rates of smoking and alcohol consumption, and their general lifestyle is health-conscious, taking the opportunity to exercise (gardening and walking), eat a healthy diet, and monitor their weight (Victor, 1991). With increasing age, people become more aware of health-maintenance. They are more likely to seek medical advice at an earlier stage than they used to, and comply more vigilantly with medical advice and treatments. They also cope with illness better than younger adults (Rodin and Salovey, 1989). Chronic illness is more frequent for the over sixty-fives and the cost to the National Health Service for each individual increases with age. Figures for 1983 approximated expenditure to be £125 per young adult, rising to £1000 for each person over the age of seventy-five years (Grundy, 1989). These kinds of statistics help fuel public debates on policy issues affecting the elderly and reflect people's concerns that the ageing population is depleting the economic base of the general population.

Once in hospital, an older person receives a lower quality service compared to anyone else. For example, Sudnow (1967) found that they had a less thorough examination when admitted into an accident and emergency department, and that they are more readily certified 'dead on arrival' compared to younger groups.

The Help The Aged Dignity on the Ward campaign encourages older people, carers and relatives to share their experiences of care within NHS provisions, many of which show how powerless they are while receiving a service. A few examples include:

> *After my mother had been on the ward for about two weeks her 'named nurse' refused to give me any information regarding a doctor's report, saying she could only inform the patient herself. The fact that my mother was eighty-five years old, in an advanced state of dementia with*

Parkinson's and I was shown as her next of kin made no difference.

My mother had short-term memory loss and we told the nurses and doctors this and it was no good telling her a thing because she had no idea what they were on about, so would they tell us, they never took any notice.

We managed to see the senior ward doctor. Tired though he was, we did not expect him to tell us so directly that Mum was 'old, has dementia, will not get any better and needs to go into care'.

(RCN, 2000a)

Examples of inequality in care provision for the older adult can also be found in community health services. Syson-Nibbs (2000), a carer for her father diagnosed with cancer, and her husband, diagnosed with dementia, compared the care given for a typically older person's disease to a physical illness that could affect someone of any age. The support of the multi-agency team for the person with cancer was far superior to that available for her husband's needs with dementia.

Ageist rationing by GPs has been highlighted through a survey conducted by Jheeta (2001). The survey of GPs found them reluctant to provide anything other than general care for patients with dementia because there is no cure, and they found it difficult to justify using scarce resources.

Elderly people do not appear to help themselves as a group, by agreeing to the negative descriptions younger people give to them. For example, Kuypers and Bengston (1973) found that the older adults shared the view that they as a group were, 'stubborn', 'touchy', 'bossy', 'incompetent', 'dependent', 'passive', 'rigid', 'irritable', 'inactive', 'withdrawn', 'suspicious', and 'indolent'.

The vast imbalance in power between the older adult and the health service needs to be addressed. This can be approached from two angles: the older adult needs to empower themselves, increasing their self-esteem and self-worth, while the rest of the population reflect on their beliefs and behaviours and facilitate the transition. Although a long way from the full authority and prestige that used to be accorded to the 'elders', the older person is already making a gradual comeback. In America, older people have acquired significant political influence as a powerful political lobby. They have done this through joining together to form groups such as the Gray Panthers and asserting themselves, rather than waiting for the younger generations to change their attitudes towards them. This approach has been shown to be particularly effective when directed at institutions such as the health services. Similar developments are now being seen in the UK.

Simple changes could be implemented by health workers to redress the balance of power between the older adult patient and the system. A person suffering from dementia may still have a preference on how they wish to be addressed. By using their preferred name, the health professional will show respect, increasing the self-worth of the individual. Nursing staff should ensure that the confused person continues to be dressed in their own clothes, and has their belongings around them to help them with their self-identity, orientation and relationships to others (RCN, 2000b).

There is a role for healthcare professionals to facilitate support groups for the older adult diagnosed with dementia, to maintain and develop their feelings of self-worth, as although very useful to the carers, support groups exclusively for carers send a strong devaluing message to the sufferer themselves. Keady and Gilliard (1999) found that early diagnosed Alzheimer's sufferers believed that they lacked; information about the disease and services available, practical help to assist their carers, and support in overcoming their anxieties.

Within the caring professions, there is a preference to work with younger adults and children rather than the elderly (Palmore, 1977).

Recruiting staff to work with the older patient is a major problem. Managers have had to be creative in the way they staff these areas within hospitals, consequently advertisements for jobs have, for a long time, offered flexibility in working hours and perks in an attempt to entice the worker.

Psychologists attempting to redress the problem of ageism by presenting the positive image of older age, can themselves be seen as ageist if they promote the continuation of middle-aged behaviour. They are assuming that middle-aged behaviour is superior to old-age behaviour and continue to perpetuate the young is best attitude.

A positive intervention for a psychologist would be to aid individuals through a successful adaptation to older life (Rowe and Kahn, 1997). They divide this process into three components:

1.   Low probability of disease and disease related disability.
2.   High cognitive and physical functional capacity.
3.   Active engagement with life.

The first component needs to be addressed when a person is young, as they need to be aware of the affects that their lifestyle will have upon their later life in terms of health. This then gives each individual the chance to make an informed choice. As this is related more to education in earlier life, it would perhaps not be seen as the role of the psychologist, but more of a teacher's role.

Maximising cognitive function by helping older people relearn or remember techniques for problem-solving and memory could be very useful, along with any therapy that increases an individual's feelings of self-worth, self-esteem, and enables them to be happy with their new, post-retirement self-concept. With the acceptance of old age can come the opportunity to assert one's self upon the community, be seen as a person and contradict stereotypical images, aiming to change local attitude.

Psychologists, along with other health workers, could also work with the elderly who have dementia and their carers to ensure the maximisation and maintenance of the older persons' skills, and helping the carer to manage, understand and adjust to the increasingly dependent parent. With an understanding of dementia, help in the practicalities of care, developing coping strategies for the carers, ie. relaxation, stress management, encouraging discussion at, for example, carer support groups, the carers are more likely to be able to cope with an ageing parent and to promote positive aspects of ageing. It may help them with their concept of ageing, and aid their adjustment to old age when they reach it. The effects of the health worker could then be seen to run through the family, extending outwards and through the generations as the change in attitude is promoted.

Attitude change could be seen as the most influential way to eradicate ageism. This should be aimed at both young and old people.

Work with the elderly could include such 'therapies' as encouraging a healthy level of reminiscence in order for the person to acknowledge good and bad in their life, to identify achievement and come to terms with 'failures', and to facilitate the moving on into another positive period in their life. This could involve identifying areas of dissatisfaction and working towards a solution, for example, if a person had a goal they had not achieved then to aid them in achieving it, or if something cannot be solved, then the psychologist can help the individual accept the situation and adjust to it.

Adjustment to life after a spouse has died is another role for the psychologist, particularly if the person has become stuck in the grieving process.

If elderly people have a much more positive opinion of themselves as a group, they may well contribute to the realisation of younger people that old age is not necessarily bad. The elderly may then get more satisfaction out of their later years through feeling better about themselves and others having a better attitude towards them.

Some aspects of ageism may be understood, but never justified. When something is understood there is a grounding on which to work to eradicate it. As with sexism and racism, there should be a positive attitude towards older people and the concept of valuing diversity should be adopted by all.

Key points

⌘ Ageing is seen as a negative process of decay in terms of a person's physical, psychological, social and economic potential and therefore one's value to society diminishes as one becomes older.

⌘ Stereotyped thinking towards older people exists within the professional arena despite being acknowledged as a target for change in many government documents. These conceptual elements of pre-justice for older people are translated into action in many instances, resulting in a reduction in the quality of services provided and less participation in their organisation.

⌘ The power-base in health is not democratic and rests with the young to determine how and where power should be shared.

⌘ The adaptation to older life should incorporate an active engagement with life itself, which will assist cognitive, physical, emotional and spiritual functioning. In turn, choice and self-determination will naturally follow.

References

Atchley RC (1985) *Social Forces and Aging.* 4th edn. Wadsworth, Belmont

Block MR, Davidson JL, Grambs JD (1981) *Women over forty: Visions and Realities.* Springer, New York

Brown J (1985) *In her Prime.* Bergin and Garvey, Massachusetts

Butler RN (1969) Age-ism: another form of bigotry. *Gerontologist* **9**: 243–6

Butler RN, Lewis MI (1977) *Aging and Mental Health.* CV Mosby, St. Louis

Coombes R (1999a) The Age of Discontent. *Nurs Times* **95**(35): 15

Coombes R (1999b) Meet Helen, 77: supportive, caring, efficient. *Nurs Times* **9**(9): 6

Grundy E (1989) Longitudinal Perspectives on the Living arrangements of the Elderly. In: Jefferys M, ed. *Growing Old in the Twentieth Century*. Routledge, London

Gutmann D (1985) The cross-cultural perspective: notes toward a comparative psychology of aging. In: Binstock RH, Shanas RH, eds. *Handbook of Aging and the Social Sciences*. 2nd edn. Van Nostrand Reinhold, New York

Jheeta K (2001) All in the mind. *Nurs Times* **97**(9): 27

Keady J, Gilliard J (1999) The early experience of Alzheimer's disease: Implications for partnership and practice. In Adams T, Clarke CL, eds. *Dementia Care: Developing Partnerships in Practice*. Baillière Tindall, London

Kuypers JA, Bengston VL (1973) Social breakdown and competence: A model of normal ageing. *Hum Development* **16**: 181–201

NHS Executive (1999) *The Diversity in Employment Code of Practice*. DfEE, Nottingham

Northcott H (1975) Too young, too old — age in the world of television. *Gerontologist* **15**: 184–6

Nuessel FH (1982) The language of ageism. *Gerontologist* **22**: 273–76

Palmore E (1990) *Ageism: Negative and Positive*. Springer, New York

Palmore E (1986) Trends in the health of the aged. *Gerontologist* **26**(3): 298– 302

Palmore E (1977) *Normal Aging*. Duke University Press, Durham, NC

Pratt F (1981) *What's it all About?* Department of Education (ERIC Document Reproductive Service No. ED 211 405), Washington, DC

Riley MW (1987) On the significance of age in society. *Am Sociological Rev* **52**: 25–7

Rodin J, Salovey P (1989) Health Psychology. *Annu Rev Psychol* **40**: 533–79

Rowe JW, Kahn RL (1997) Successful ageing. *Gerontologist* **37**(4): 433–9

Royal College of Nursing (2000a) online at: http://www.rcn.org.uk/dementia/say.html

Royal College of Nursing (2000b) online at: http://www.rcn.org.uk/dementia/learn.html

Seefeldt C (1989) Intergenerational programmes: impact on attitudes. *Haworth Journal*: 185–93

Soldo BJ, Manton KG (1983) Health status and service needs of the oldest old: current patterns and future trends. *Milbank Memorial Fund Quarterly – Health and Society* **63**(2): 286–319

Stokes G(1995) *On being old: The psychology of later life*. The Falmer Press, Washington DC

Sudnow D (1967) *Passing on: The social organisation of dying*. Prentice-Hall, London

Syson-Nibbs I (2000) Alzheimer's: dispelling the myths (a personal view). *Elderly Care* **11**(10): 16–18

Traxler AJ (1980) *Let's get Gerontologized: Developing a Sensitivity to Aging. The Multi-purpose Senior Centre Concept: A Training Manual for Practitioners Working with the Aging*. Illinois Department of Aging, Springfield, IL

Victor CR (1991) *Health and Health Care in Later Life*. Open University Press, Milton Keynes

10

Psychiatry and power

Deenesh Khoosal

Introduction

The medical profession is considered to be a powerful discipline, not only because it has been around for hundreds of years but also because it deals with a subject that concerns all of us, namely, life itself. Doctors have a high rating for trustworthiness despite recent adverse publicity following the Bristol and Shipman enquiries. Most medical practitioners are respected for their altruism and their influence often extends into matters well beyond their professional training.

Despite their own adverse publicity, disciplines allied to medicine such as nursing, midwifery, psychology and paramedics, also enjoy a similarly high public regard. These professionals, however, do not have as strong a 'power base'. For instance, the influence of psychologists is hampered because psychology as a profession has not been around long enough. The effect of this can be far reaching, for example, some health insurers in Britain require private psychological treatments to be pre-authorised by a psychiatrist.

Psychiatrists, as specialist medical practitioners, enjoy almost the same power base as their non-psychiatric medical colleagues. Only 'almost' because psychiatry is regarded by some as the 'Cinderella' of the medical profession, and has not been afforded the resources of other medical specialities. Hard working mental health charities also suffer a similar fate, as they do not succeed in raising as much money as charities for cancer research and children's health. These tend to be at the top of the 'charity league' table as far as fund-raising and public awareness is concerned. Fear and stigma may have something to do with this.

Psychiatry exerts its influence and power well beyond a purely 'medical model' fashioned as it is by many influences including anthropology, sociology, pharmacology, theology and philosophy. Quality psychopharmacological research has brought innovative, safer treatments that have revolutionised the management of many psychiatric disorders. Already products such as Prozac have become household names with a website, songs and even books about it. Prozac's place in history is assured because it is the only antidepressant in the handful of drugs that has generated a $1 billion sale figure for its manufacturer. All this will extend the influence and power of psychiatry just as these fields in turn are strengthened in almost a symbiotic way.

Medical treatments in the past, such as leeches for dropsy and red-hot pokers for haemorrhoids are no longer used. Psychiatry has also had its share of treatments that would not now be regarded as beneficial, such as insulin, coma and workhouses. None of these are used nowadays. The need to be scientific and evidence based will help to remove the undeserved stigma associated with the practice of psychiatry. We are aware that this is happening, as there is a greater willingness to seek help earlier for mental health problems. We are already seeing a more informed doctor/patient relationship develop. This will undoubtedly promote earlier access to health which will, in turn, strengthen psychiatry.

Background

Psychiatry in a setting of power

It is estimated that in the UK six million people are diagnosed as having mental illness each year, and that one in four of the population suffers from some degree of mental or emotional distress (Mental Health Foundation, 1990). This represents a healthcare problem affecting many more people than cancer or Aids and accounts for £2 billion of the NHS budget alone. Not all sufferers will seek help, nor can the current system cope should all of these sufferers present for help. The potential demand is, however, enormous.

The powerful images of institutional psychiatry documented by Goffman (1961), and immortalised in celluloid by Jack Nicholson in *One Flew Over the Cuckoo's Nest* remain as a lasting testimony to the abuse of power for many people. That this should have occurred at all is a grim reminder that some people working in these institutions did usurp power for themselves. This was totally unacceptable. The thrust to community care kindled by Enoch Powell's famous 'water towers over the horizon' speech (Hall and Brockington, 1991) led to the ultimate demise of many of the Victorian asylums with their inbuilt potential for abuse. The move to community care has largely been achieved but only after many government reports were issued (Khoosal and Jones, 1989; 1990–1991). Community care is perceived as being relatively free of the abuse of power, based as it is within the community which shares power through partnership arrangements with service providers.

Some would argue that the pendulum has swung back too far now as care is compromised by too few available hospital beds (Office for Health Economics [OHE], 1997). Community care, while having the distinct advantage of being able to treat an individual within his familiar environment, often with the assistance of specific intervention measures, such as assertive outreach and home treatment (Marks, 1994), cannot always care for those people who are severely mentally ill. Sometimes there is no alternative to hospitalisation, although smaller purpose built in-patient facilities attached to a community mental health team base are valued most.

Mental Health Act

A further battleground for power struggles is enshrined in the Mental Health Act. This allows for the compulsory admission, detention and treatment of people with mental health problems who are unwilling or unable to accept psychiatric management because of their mental illness. The legal provisions to do this are clearly outlined in this Act so that abuse of power is prevented while attempting at the same time to balance the civil liberty of the patient and that of society.

The Mental Health Act of 1959 was not considered to be appropriate for the latter part of the twentieth century, as the public perception of mental illness had changed. The Mental Health Act 1983 replaced it. It owes much of its statute to civil libertarians such as Larry Gostin (Khoosal, 1983; Bowden, 1995). This Act now governs compulsory admission, detention and treatment. A further reform of the 1983 Act has been mooted following several homicides by psychiatric patients which have captured public imagination (Bowden, 1995). The work on this is reaching completion though complex issues relating to treatability of personality disorder and compulsory treatment in the community, have generated much debate within the profession itself.

The legislation that was introduced in 1983 to prevent abuse of power by psychiatrists concerns the right of patients to appeal against detention to the managers of the hospital and/or the mental health review tribunals. This was regarded as being ground breaking then but is now accepted as good clinical practice. The Mental Health Act Commission was also established. This independent body has wide powers in 'policing' the 1983 Mental Health Act and has never hesitated to perform its legitimate function. The safeguard of this external scrutiny guarantees that psychiatric practice is not brought into disrepute through any misuse of delegated statutory power. No one knows what the revised Act will contain for certain, but it is unlikely that the twin principles of delegating responsibility for compulsory detention while regulating power at the same time will be compromised.

Terminology

The need for clear definition in any field is essential for obvious reasons. This is especially true for a discipline such as psychiatry, functioning as it does at several interfaces such as the mind, brain, meaning, understanding, etc. all at the same time. All of these have their own definitions that may be of specific relevance to psychiatry. The demand for clear terminology in mental health is driven by stigma against value loaded terms of the past such as 'moron', which were symbolic of abuse.

Patients, too, prefer to be referred to as 'clients' or 'users', though some prefer 'survivors' which reflects their experience of services. It is not difficult to see the backdrop for this (Hodgkiss, 2000). In addition, the abuse of psychiatry for political purposes is well documented by authors like Solzhenitsyn in *The Gulag Archipelago*. Abuse has occurred in many countries over many years but must be guarded against, as it can never be condoned. Emerging relatively unscathed through one of these systems is, indeed, a survival experience. Most British psychiatrists would be rightly appalled if such blatant abuse took place, but the distinction can be blurred if more subtle manipulation were to take place.

Alternative explanations to help understand these experiences have been sought over the years. Foremost among these is the anti-psychiatry movement led by people such as Laing (1960). These exponents have made a distinct impact on users, carers and informed professionals. The legacy of this movement is a reminder that views which are alternative to conventional ones do exist and enrich the practice of psychiatry through their very diversity. As long as psychiatrists continue to acknowledge these different opinions and to shape practice accordingly, the potential for abuse will be minimised.

Risk indicators and vulnerable groups

It is clear that mental health disorders occur throughout the population. Certain factors are linked to a higher incidence of mental illness, putting some people at greater risk. Labelling or stereotyping these people may make service providers think that they are doing something, but this is not so. They need instead to concentrate on developing active dialogue with these groups. This will help identify vulnerability factors so that appropriate action to minimise risk can be taken.

Social factors

Social factors such as deprivation, poor housing, financial hardship and unemployment, are known to contribute to the development of mental ill health (Holmes *et al*, 1944; Rigg, 1993). Mental ill health can in turn magnify the exposure to these adverse social factors, either through disability or stigma. The power to resolve adverse social factors lies more in Westminster than in psychiatric clinics where the adverse effect of policy decisions is seen most. It is the psychiatric team which is often left to fight for services for their vulnerable patients. This is a good example of the constructive use of the power vested in psychiatry.

Women

Women are at a greater risk of developing mental illness than men. One in three women present to their general practitioner with some degree of psychiatric morbidity compared to men who present at the rate of one in four. It is known that 10% of women suffer from depressive illness. This is twice as many as men. In urban working class communities this figure can rise to 20% among women with children at home (Taylor and Taylor, 1989). Women are more likely to be admitted to psychiatric hospitals, are more likely to be prescribed medication, are more likely to be unhappy with the quality of information available and with the choice of treatment. Hardly surprisingly, women feel disenfranchised by psychiatry and the power they see vested in it. It is important that women are involved in identifying their own needs and ensure that initiatives that actually address their needs are supported. At the Bristol Cancer Help Centre, a holistic approach has arisen with a re-distribution and sharing of power with impressive outcomes. This is a good example of harnessing the existing power of each individual for a common good.

Age

Increasing age is linked to the prevalence of infirmity and dementia that affects one in five of the eighty-five plus age group (Melzer, 1992). The effect of social factors such as isolation, reduced income, bereavement, etc. can be more profound on the elderly. Elderly people also tend to be less forthcoming in taking an active role as consumers of care services and need special consideration. Integrated multi-disciplinary and multi-agency approaches will best meet the needs of this vulnerable group. Where this takes place, eg. the NAVJIVAN project in Leicester, a quality service much appreciated by its users has developed. This is a good example of how to succeed better in co-ordinating the power within existing services.

Homelessness

It is clear that homeless people suffer from higher levels of psychiatric morbidity than the general population. Mental illness may either be a cause or a consequence of homelessness. Mental illness is also likely to worsen with continued homelessness (Lamb and Lamb, 1990). Engaging this population is the challenge for this decade. For example, schizophrenia affects 30–50% of homeless people while alcohol abuse is also three to five times more prevalent. Poorly planned discharges from acute service can contribute considerably to the perpetuation of homelessness. If the root causes of homelessness were to be adequately addressed, this dis-enfranchised group of people can once again integrate within mainstream society with all its implications. Should this take place, it would be a good example of returning power to the powerless.

Children and adolescents

This group undoubtedly has special needs as some 10% of children and adolescents suffer from emotional and behavioural disorders that produce disability in about 2% of cases (Office of Population Censuses and Surveys [OPCS], 1989). Physical and sexual abuse, learning disabilities and severe physical disabilities are further risk factors for children and adolescents. Psychiatrists working with this client group traditionally involve families in service delivery. This has been a constructive working pattern. The Children's Act imposes further clear obligations requiring sharing of information. This will prevent battlelines being drawn and assist in the continuation of good practise. This is a good example of what can be achieved through power sharing.

Black and minority ethnic groups

Even though British society today has been enriched by diverse multicultural influences, the battle for power is most evident in services for users from black and other minority ethnic groups. These groups report being the victims of a 'double whammy' — abused by psychiatry (like all the other groups) but also being subjected to racism at the same time.

The reasons for this are that:

❖ People from black and other minority ethnic groups are marginalised when it comes to health provision. As a result, disengagement with poorly designed services takes place especially for those most in need, ending in a greater use of the Mental Health Act for vulnerable people.

❖ Black and other minority ethnic groups may be subjected to discrimination in the treatment received for mental health problems (Balrajan and Raleigh, 1993). Physical treatments such as medication are made available more often than talking therapies such as psychotherapy.

❖ African-Caribbean people tend to be diagnosed as suffering from schizophrenia and other serious psychiatric illnesses and given higher doses of medication more often than any other cultural group (Soni, 1995).

❖ African-Caribbean people are more likely to be subjected to the Mental Health Act, to be taken to a place of safety and to be over-represented in forensic services and in locked wards (Davies *et al,* 1998).

❖ Asian people tend to have similar rates of psychiatric morbidity as the indigenous population. However, concerns are raised for the much higher suicide rates for young Asian women when compared to the national average (Soni, 1996).

Racism

Many reasons are put forward for this state of affairs. Racism is very high on the list. Institutional racism is now acknowledged to exist by the McPherson Report following the Lawrence enquiry even though there has been no doubt about its existence in the NHS for some time (Commission for Racial Equality [CRE], 1996; Beishon *et al,* 1995). Workers from black and other minority ethnic groups report experiencing racism in everyday professional work in addition to institutional racism. Those workers are baffled by this but feel helpless, as institutions are not well known for taking up the cudgels on their behalf. Accusations of 'imagining racism' or having a 'chip on the shoulder' and being branded as a 'trouble maker' are not unusual.

Existing service structures, service delivery models and consultation exercises by whatever name are viewed by black users with suspicion. Users have had expectations raised with reports produced by people who then moved up the promotion ladder without effecting change so that users feel used. Users from black and other minority ethnic groups are able to identify individuals who abuse their power, are covertly racist and disabling. Faced with this past experience, it is no wonder that people from black and other minority ethnic groups are understandably suspicious of statutory services. The abuse of power then becomes a corporate issue with little perceived prospect of change by this group of disadvantaged people.

Coping strategies

Black and other minority ethnic groups have ended up developing their own services wherever possible often with little help or support from the statutory agencies. Organisations such as Asian Counselling

Services (Leicester), Share in Maudsley Black Action (SIMBA, London), Chinese Mental Health Association, and Voice shared concern about this. These organisations are not afraid to let their views be known about what is actually happening, especially regarding gaps in service. Emphasis has dwelt on power sharing through empowerment and advocacy models to achieve progress.

It is evident that the different ethnic groups require specific rather than homogenous targeting. Special needs within particular groups also need to be addressed separately, such as the needs of women. This should be the basis of all user consultation exercises so that active input into decision-making processes takes place from the outset. There is hope that things will change as long as these voices are heard at the highest level. Open consultation exercises with inbuilt planned monitoring and evaluation of developments will meet the needs of black and other minority ethnic groups. To succeed, there must be cultural sensitivity in interactions with people and cultural competency in the therapies available. This is the only way that power share will provide services valued by the users themselves. This is a good example of providing what users want in a true power sharing process.

The way forward

Areas in which issues related to power could potentially be problematic have been reviewed in relation to medicine but with specific emphasis on psychiatry. While the issues are clear, the solutions are less so. Universal prescriptive solutions do not exist as local factors and local users must determine outcome. This improves the prospect of services, recovery, and the use of patient opinion as an audit tool. The latter is valuable even though it does not always support the care providers think their clients want. The spate of documents from the Department of Health and the Government, including the recent National Service Framework, are testimony to the commitment to encourage meaningful involvement of users and carers (NHS Executive, 1994; DoH, 1999). The role of users has now been highlighted in an unambiguous way. Users do have rights as well as responsibilities. They are entitled to be consulted and to influence service provision.

Service development

User participation in the development of strategy and in-service evaluation should take account of people with particular or specific needs in accessing mental health care. Building on existing user groups and local networks is an obvious first step. This starts by noting what actually exists in the community and then by encouraging the development and continuation of user groups. The role of individuals in groups may change from time to time perhaps due even to a relapse of illness but this should not be an excuse for non-involvement. Agencies need to make services user-friendly and equitable by firmly placing users centrally in all mental health matters.

Involving more than one service user wherever possible to join committees and working parties is less daunting and will provide a wider range of opinions. Scheduling meetings at a time and place convenient for users, followed by a true record of the minutes will also encourage participation. Jargon-free explanations of how to get issues onto the agenda and how the process of decision making operates will help. This process may initially seem intimidating but once the legitimate concerns of users are acknowledged, it is always surprising to discover just how much common ground exists and how much improvement can be achieved with equal partnerships.

Honesty is vital at all times. Promising only what can be delivered prevents frustration, disillusionment and charges of 'tokenism'. Trust will be encouraged if specific issues producing quick results are addressed first. Regular feedback on progress is needed for the process to continue. All this can be facilitated by publicity in different languages, taking on cultural issues, and meeting specific needs such as those of women as appropriate. A healthy outcome would be for a two-way process to develop which informs users about psychiatry and for the statutory agencies to learn as well. Active consultation with users in the community is the only way to stimulate their contribution to planning and service development. By doing this, the service will be valued by users and providers alike, so that the concept of power sharing becomes meaningful.

User involvement

The user involvement movement arose from the experience of psychiatry by its recipients. Users have increasingly been challenging and resisting disempowerment by speaking out against the existing system and by working towards the development of alternatives (Fernando, 1995).

Users of mental health services and their advocates should have access to the fullest information about their condition, treatment and possible treatments, information about medication and outcomes. Information should be expressed in language and terminology that users can understand. Interpreter services can be of particular value in this situation. It cannot be over-emphasised that it is not appropriate to use relatives for interpreting.

Users must be made aware of statutory, non-statutory and out-of-hours emergency services that are available to them, and how to access them. Users who are subject to the Mental Health Act (1983) have special requirements. They must have information about their rights, how to make a complaint, how to obtain representation and how to seek advocacy. The outreach and key worker systems can work well especially if the carer is also informed of the name and number of this person. Users and their carers need time and space to discuss and express their feelings about their illness and this needs to be facilitated.

Assumptions should never be made about what users want from the service. Users and their carers will say what is on their mind given the opportunity. This is of particular importance in our multi-cultural society. It is only by fully involving users that sharing of power can proceed constructively.

Advocacy

Advocacy is defined as, 'people promoting the rights of themselves or others' (Read and Wallcraft, 1994). The advocate's role is to support the user and to reflect the user's wishes. Individual users are entitled to have their views and wishes considered when care for them is planned. Should users find this hard to do, they should have the services of an advocate do this for them.

Better care can be planned when ample notice is given of a review of a user's care plan so that friends, relatives or advocates can be invited. The user must express his view and be permitted to change his mind about the care plan without fear of recrimination. The user's key worker could act as advocate if one is needed and if no other advocate is present. Staff members, acting as advocates, may have divided loyalties and be unable to represent the client's interest impartially. The advocate should, wherever possible, be independent from both the care agency and the user's family. Advocacy should be an important part of good clinical practice.

Empowerment

The empowerment model usually equates to regaining control of one's own life even though differences both in cultural and political terms exist about what empowerment means in practice. Empowerment of black users can be either reactive (the response to the impact of inequality upon people's lives) or innovative (initiatives to enable black people to exercise greater control over their own psychiatric management). Empowerment models must be able to co-exist with beliefs and traditions fundamental to a culture. This will achieve success within it rather than at its margins only.

The experience of having control taken away by psychiatry to some extent unites the disparate collection of people who use mental health services. Nonetheless, the essential ingredients of empowerment include users campaigning for changes in the psychiatric system via action groups, user involvement on planning and development committees with service providers, promoting alternative inter-pretation of emotional distress and encouraging more appropriate survivor-led support. User empowerment requires a commitment to staff training and development. Thus, effective user empowerment initiatives require real investment in people and facilities.

Issues relating to who decides what is empowering for an individual or group and how to deal with the effects of the psychiatric system on users remain pertinent even now. The motivation to get something done initially arose from the sense of despair and anger about the injustices seen in the treatment of black people by black workers who became concerned about the plight of their particular community. Black users have now taken this on board.

Information and training

A clear strategy for providing users with information needs to be in place. Staff responsible for implementation need to be identified and a clear timetable for action should be made available. A fully funded strategy for multi-agency collaboration should also be in place. The responsibility of each agency should be explicit to make this successful. A clear strategy for training staff in these matters needs to be in place. The role of service users in training staff must never be ignored. The commitment of all healthcare staff needs to be confirmed to make the whole system work. Appropriate training in cultural sensitivity in their interactions with people and cultural competency in the therapies available underpins the whole problem.

Cost implications arise in developing consumer participation programmes in any area of health care. Ring-fenced resources need to be allocated for information leaflets in different languages, for office space, for staff participation and training, for user/carer workshops and for paying users for their time commitment to make this process successful.

Complaints

Most of the time, most things go well for most people but it is inevitable that things occasionally go wrong even in the best of services. This may result in a complaint. There should be no hesitation in advising users about their right to complain, how to obtain a second opinion and how to access the complaint procedure. All staff should be familiar with the complaints procedure and their role within it. Involving users in the development of a complaints procedure at the outset will ensure that it is accessible. Progress regarding investigation of the complaint and prompt feedback after investigation will ensure that the complaint is handled sympathetically, even if it has no substance.

A culture of seeing complaints as a constructive feedback process rather than criticism of individuals or the system, needs to be inculcated. It is not unknown for providers to use complaints to improve facilities and even earmark resources for specific purposes, such as staff training. The process is not completed without the monitoring of complaints as part of the strategic information gathering system. This information should be collated and made available to users and providers to promote full sharing of power.

Monitoring/evaluation/audit

It is essential to monitor, evaluate and audit user involvement to ensure that what is intended takes place. Evidence should be independently sought so that users have appropriate information readily available, access to an advocate and the opportunity to exercise choice in their own care plans. User satisfaction with the service at all levels should be ascertained as well. The complaints procedure may be informative to this end. The acquisition of user views and audits of their satisfaction are key to the development of services, with the number of complaints being a key indicator: user groups and independent advocates are essential to sustain the quality of services. Users must also have a real say in evaluating these outcomes. Audit is the tool by which this occurs. There is much to commend this process no matter how anxiety provoking it may seem initially. After all, the service is for the users themselves and service providers ignore this at their peril.

Conclusion

In the past, power within psychiatry was retained by professionals. They were considered to know what was best for service users. This led to a system that users did not value. They are now saying that those services were not always appropriate to their needs. They do not want this to continue, especially as considerable change is taking place in legislation and in the public's perception of mental health.

The voice of users has grown louder with insistence that things need to change meaningfully if real progress is to be made. User involvement through strategies such as empowerment, advocacy, consultancy and participation seems logical and overdue. This movement has now made its debut despite professional fear of the unknown and users' fear of being abused once again by the very system they aim to change.

There is real hope for change. Prejudices on both sides, though understandable, have no place in today's mental health service provision. A better understanding of each other's perspective and a willingness to work together will provide better health for all. The best user-friendly services can be made available by doing just this.

Much has changed for the better already. Much more is changing even now and it is likely that the rest will change in the near future. Good models of care already exist so there is nothing to fear. Some paths to achieve these changes have been reviewed and must be considered seriously if further progress is to be made. Achieving this will enhance services for all, but especially for those for whom the service is designed — the users and carers themselves. There can be little doubt that this will achieve the equalisation of power in psychiatry.

Key points

⌘ Psychiatry is influenced by anthropology, sociology, pharmacology, theology and philosophy. It adapts with changes in society and reflects the context in which it occurs.

⌘ Psychiatry has developed an opinion that touches every element of society, yet without agreement from those outside its boundaries it cannot exist. (A psychiatrist without a patient becomes redundant.)

⌘ Psychiatry has been blamed for the perpetuation of oppression in the past, however, it is good intentioned by law and is striving to do better.

⌘ Psychiatrists are increasingly willing to enable user participation to influence the type of care prescribed, however, ultimate responsibility for decisions will always shape the extent to which this can be achieved.

⌘ Prejudice has no place in contemporary mental health care, and it is everyone's responsibility to work together to share the available power.

References

Balrajan R, Raleigh SV (1993) *Ethnicity and Health — A Guide for the NHS.* Department of Health, London

Beishon S, Virdee S, Hagell A (1995) *Nursing in a Multi-Ethnic NHS.* Policy Studies Institute, London

Bowden P (1995) Confidential Inquiry into Homicides and Suicides by Mentally Ill People. A Preliminary Report on Homicide. *Psychiatr Bull Roy Coll Psychiatrists* **19**: 65

Commision for Racial Equality (1996) *Appointing NHS Consultants and Senior Registrars.* CRE, London

Davies EA (1998) British Psychiatric Morbidity. *Br J Psychiatry* **173**: 4–7

Department of Health (1999) *National Service Framework — Mental Health.* DoH, London

Fernando S, ed (1995) *Mental Health in a Multi-Ethnic Society.* Routledge, London

Goffman E (1961) *Asylums: Essays on social situation of mental patients and other inmates.* 9th edn. Penguin Books, Harmondsworth

Hall P, Brockington IF, eds (1991) *The Closure of Mental Hospitals.* Gaskell, London

Hodgkiss A (2000) User, client or patient: What do you call people receiving treatment for mental health problems? *Psychiatr Bull* **24**: 441

Holmes SP, Jenner D, Barnes SB (1944) *The Trent Health Gain Investigation Programme for People with Mental Health Problems* (Part I). Sheffield Trent Regional Health Authority, Sheffield

Hupperd FA, Roth M, Gore M (1987) *Health and Lifestyle Survey — a Preliminary Report.* Health Promotions Research Trust, London

Khoosal DI (1983) The Mental Health Act (Amendment) Bill — an Oxford Conference. *Psychiatr Bull Roy Coll Psychiatrists* **27**: 15.

Khoosal DI, Jones PH (1989) Community care again: a need for action. *Community Care J Roy Soc Med* **82**: 451–2

Khoosal DI, Jones PH (1990–1991)Worcester Development Project — Where do patients go when hospitals close? *Health Trends* **22**(4): 137–41

Laing RD (1960) *The Divided Self.* Pelican, London

Lamb R, Lamb D (1990) Factors contributing to homelessness amongst the chronically and severely mentally ill. *Hospital and Community Psychiatry* **41**: 301–5

Marks IM (1994) Home-based versus hospital-based care for serious mental illness. *Br J Psychiatry* **165**: 179–94

Mental Health Foundation (1990) *Mental Illness: The Fundamental Facts.* Mental Health Foundation, London

Melzer D (1992) *Dementia.* NHS Management Executive, London

NHS Executive (1994) *Focus on User Empowerment in Mental Health Care NHS Executive.* Trent Regional Health Authority, Trent

Office for Health Economics (1997) *Compendium of Health Statistics.* OHE, London

Office of Population Censuses and Surveys (1989) *The Prevalence of Disability among Children.* OPCS, London

Read AJ, Wallcraft J (1994) *Guidelines and Advocacy for Mental Health Workers.* Unison/MIND, London

Rigg EM (1993) Sharing power. In: *Involving Patients and Consumers.* Health Service Journal — Health Management Guide

Soni R (1995) *Mental Health in Black and Minority Ethnic People: The Fundamental Facts.* The Mental Health Foundation, London

Soni R (1996) Suicide Patterns and Trends in People of Indian Sub-Continent and Caribbean Origin in England and Wales. *Ethn Health* **1**: 15–63

Taylor J, Taylor D (1989) *Mental Health in the 1990s — From Custody to Care?* Office of Health Economics, London

11

Empowerment in forensic mental health: the challenge to leaders

Ray Rowden

I first entered nursing in 1970 as a pre-nursing student at St Augustine's Hospital, a 1600-bedded institution in Kent. I vividly remember my early experiences. I worked on a ward for seventy-seven elderly men; half were incontinent, most chronically institutionalised. The beds were arrayed in long and rigid straight lines. On entering the dormitory at 6.30 am, our first job was to wake patients, in a stench of urine. The patients who were less able were handled roughly, like lumps of meat. One flannel and the same water were used to clean all who were less mobile. No screens or privacy were part of this regime; the task was to get the patients up as quickly as possible and into a vast day room.

The patients had a miserable and boring existence, their day punctuated only by meals and the rigid routine imposed by a rotten system. There was one bathroom for these seventy-seven souls with only two baths. From Monday to Saturday, there were rostered bath days to fit all the patients in, essentially a conveyor belt with no privacy. Anyone incontinent would be wheeled on a commode and hosed down in the sluice area. Patients were routinely put on commodes in the day area or a passage just off it, in full view of one another and the rest of the ward.

On a Sunday, when there were no rostered baths, I got into the habit of letting some of the patients have a relaxed bath, with a cup of tea and privacy. The regular staff found this highly amusing and, as a seventeen-year-old, I was not prepared for any of this. A distinguished elderly gentleman, in the later stages of dementia, especially enjoyed his Sunday bath. About seven weeks into the profession, I took this man for his bath, made him a cup of tea and added plenty of foam and salts into his bath to make it more relaxing. He was enjoying his tea and his soak when a staff nurse entered the bathroom eating a banana and asked me in a highly inappropriate and unprofessional manner what I thought I was doing. I explained that I was giving Mr X a quiet bath. He took the half eaten fruit, rammed it in the face of the patient, forcing his head underwater. The patient was gasping for breath, with his limbs flaying in fear and water everywhere. I was frozen, but finally pulled the staff nurse off.

The staff nurse thought that this was a huge joke and went on to lecture me about what I would need to learn if I were to understand the business of mental nursing. This was really about power. It was his way of showing me the hierarchy and that he was above me and we were above the patients. I spoke to the charge nurse about the incident and was told very firmly not to make a fuss. Nothing was done, and I entered student training as a very confused person.

My three years of RMN training exposed me to further awful experiences as to how institutions treat people labelled mentally ill. The rest is history. In 1973, a contemporary of mine in training and a young nursing assistant compiled a critique of the hospital and circulated this internally. It was their attempt to ask this hospital to examine itself. The response from the hospital management was predictable. The authors were labelled as inexperienced, naïve, not understanding the nature of nursing. They were patted on the head and ignored.

They went on to annotate their document, providing dates and times of abuse and went public to the region and the media. From then on, it was all-out war. The two authors were condemned by the hierarchy, physically threatened, abusive posters were put up on notice boards, and in short, the institution closed in upon itself to protect its very being.

At this stage, a small group of younger staff, including myself, had provided details to the annotated document and we pushed for a full inquiry. The inquiry, chaired by the late Hampden-Inskip QC, eventually proved that the critique was entirely valid (South East Thames Regional Health Authority, 1974).

In the period of the inquiry I was one of the key witnesses. I received anonymous threatening phone calls, found nails in my car tyres and had faeces smeared on my front door. Other witnesses received similar or worse warnings that blowing the whistle had a cost. This period was well described by Virginia Beardshaw (Beardshaw, 1981).

I recount this experience because I find myself, at the start of a new century, questioning how much, if at all, institutional care of people with mental health needs has changed?

Since that time, I have collected a catalogue of experience in how institutions under threat protect themselves. In 1979, as a Royal College of Nursing officer in Wales, I met two students undertaking a general nursing course on a three-month psychiatric placement at Whitchurch Hospital in Cardiff. These students had observed patient abuse, and yet again, I saw the authorities try to play down the experience of the students, alleging inexperience, and again media exposure was needed to get any real action taken.

Later, in the early 1980s, we saw scandal emerging from Broadmoor Hospital following a television documentary. Depressingly, the institution tried to defend the indefensible and I had to comment in the nursing press (Rowden, 1981).

In 1986 I returned to mental health as general manager of services in West Lambeth, which included Tooting Bec Hospital, a 700-bedded institution. On arrival, I was presented with a health advisory service report (HAS, 1986).

The report provided a catalogue of shameful treatment, neglect and abuse. I found ample evidence of staff corrupting systems and evidence that the situation had gone on unchecked by authorities for years. I am pleased to say that my successors and I re-provided services and shut the place down!

Through the 1990s my repertoire was expanded as a trustee of Hamlet, a voluntary body working with survivors of psychiatric systems in central and eastern Europe. One of my first visits with Hamlet was to the Greek island of Leros in 1993, where appalling conditions had been exposed in the island's large mental hospital. On arrival, it was clear that the hospital authorities wanted our visit tightly chaperoned. A colleague and I slipped the net and talked freely to some of the nurses and assistants, and we managed to get into the wards unfettered during an afternoon and evening.

This was a European Union country in the early 1990s, yet we found patients shackled to beds, saw evidence of beatings and witnessed patients assaulting their weaker peers, unquestioned by staff. We entered one ward where the staff were asleep. We found a room locked but could hear muffled voices. We demanded the room be opened and found a blackened out space, reeking of urine and faeces. As I walked into the darkness, I was aware of hands grasping at my feet. I managed to rip down the cover at the window and found around twenty people crammed into this tiny space, with some shackled to an iron bed. These poor individuals were the forgotten fragments of a civilised and wealthy nation.

On later trips in Estonia, Romania and elsewhere, I found, and continue to find ample evidence of a similar quality. Systems which abuse people on a dramatic and terrifying scale.

In 1996, I found myself close to the three high secure hospitals in England, when appointed Director of the High Secure Psychiatric Services Commissioning Board in the NHS Executive. Here, I was supposed to remodel these hospitals into mainstream NHS frameworks and generate alternative service models. In late 1996, Ashworth Hospital had a series of abscondences, all of which had to be reported to ministers and defended. A patient submitted a dossier on Ashworth, in which he alleged security breaches, staff corruption, free availability of pornographic material and, most worryingly, of paedophile activity on a ward.

Predictably, the authorities at the hospital denied the accuracy of the testimony of this patient. The hospital attempted to cover up this dossier. Again, the rest is history; these events eventually led to the Fallon Inquiry in 1997 (DoH, 1999). In this report, it was vividly shown that the majority of testimony from this patient was accurate and the Inquiry recommended that closure of Ashworth was the only option. Some years later, Government has still not dealt with the thorny problems of Ashworth. As I write, I am aware of a patient who remains incarcerated in a high security hospital, despite the fact that independent experts and professionals at the hospital have all said that he no longer needs this level of security.

In the year 2000, as a specialist adviser to the House of Commons Select Committee on Health, I read and listened to copious amounts of evidence from users of mental health services and those who care for them informally (DoH, 2000a). The depressing theme of much of this evidence was that too often, statutory agencies and professionals simply ignore the experience of such people.

In modern Britain, in too many cases in the name of therapy, we subject vulnerable individuals to the most degrading experiences. In some secure settings, I believe we make matters worse, rather than better for people. The treatment of women and black and other minority groups in most secure settings is not far short of a national scandal.

What does this canter through thirty years of mental health services reveal about the management of such services? I am of a view that leading, planning, organising and providing these services does not get either the attention or status needed. The mad are on the margins of society (Sayce, 2000). The mad who commit serious offences are simply beyond the pale! From discussions with politicians of all parties, over many years, it is clear that there are not many votes in madness.

As a consequence, the relative position of those who choose to work within mental health is devalued at every level. Psychiatry is low status medicine, mental health nurses are perceived as not being as real as their counterparts in paediatric or general nursing, therapists with glamour are rarely found in mental health. Yet managing such services, and working within them, especially forensic services, remains one of the most complex and challenging roles in any society.

The other clear trend in abuse of mentally ill people lies in the mind-set of poor-quality staff, who view their patients as 'different' or 'apart' from them, as normal people. The abuses I have witnessed over decades happen because staff, a community, whole systems, and sometimes, whole countries, are content to view the mad as being almost sub-human, not of us and among us. How else can we explain the ability of humans to accept the clearly unacceptable on a daily basis, becoming immune to the awfulness around them? Terrifyingly, we witnessed similar processes at work in Nazi Germany, in the persecution of the Jewish Community and others. The same is at work here. We are content to put those we perceive as 'apart' in closed worlds and leave them hidden away.

The challenge facing the provider of services to people with mental health needs who offend is to strike and maintain a delicate balance between security and public safety, on the one hand, and a therapeutic regime, on the other. This has to be the toughest managerial and clinical act in the universe. It calls for skills of a high order.

A key issue underpinning the management and leadership of such services lies in the values of the organisation. How much time are managers able to grab to examine thoroughly the principles and values enthusing their teams and organisations? Yet, it is this that can guide a service well through troubled times. It must also be made explicit that these values cannot be compromised in running services. If values are well explored, defined and clearly understood, I submit that this can only enhance the therapeutic quality of a service and be a better guarantee of security for staff and patients.

Things go awry in the larger institutions because there is often a muddle concerning their values. The high secure hospitals provide a classic example of this. These hospitals are simply unclear about their overall purpose. As a result, we witness all manner of dysfunctional behaviour in these organisations.

On the one hand, staff and patients are encouraged to view the therapeutic goal as the primary task, like the rest of the NHS; on the other, they are subject to prison-like values and associated culture in publications from officialdom (DoH, 2000b). Is it any wonder that such places are confused, unmanageable and subject to crises? A wise manager will invest time in examining and clearly articulating the values of the service and will make it plain that those values are always open to robust review, but never compromised. Security is important, in a physical sense. But the highest walls, the most elaborate electronic surveillance will never replace the situational security offered to patients and staff, where therapeutic goals predominate, staff and patients communicate well and trust is built. If we learn anything at all from the Ashworth Inquiry, it is that things go gloriously wrong when values are of poor quality, are absent, or profoundly compromised.

All efforts in staff training, support and development must have the values of the service at their core and all staff need to understand this.

In the closed world of forensic mental health services, a wise manager will ensure transparency and exposure to a wide range of checks and balances. It is too easy in such services to rely simply upon the institutional framework of scrutiny. The NHS legislation, mental health law, commissioning teams, together with a plethora of other bodies and requirements, all subject forensic services to varying levels of scrutiny. This is as it should be in settings where we are depriving fellow citizens of their liberty. But is it enough?

Some forward thinking services have arranged for such scrutiny. The High Secure Psychiatric Services Commissioning Board established a user-led advisory council and some units have rigorous advocacy schemes. The emphasis must be on rigour. The *NHS Plan* (DoH, 2000c) proposes the establishment of patient advocates across the NHS. This has now happened and the challenge to forensic services will be real.

Advocacy in general healthcare, where people are in settings by way of choice, is a relatively straightforward affair. Advocacy services for patients detained against their free will is far more complex. Empowerment is a little like pregnancy — when did you last meet a woman who was half pregnant? Empowerment, like pregnancy, cannot be partial. If it is, it is not real. In many cases I have seen half-baked advocacy schemes. Too often, advocates and clients are allowed to take up the soft issues, like food or decoration. The moment such schemes challenge harder issues, like abuse or rights to information about treatment options, the organisation will run a mile.

Good advocacy is possible in such settings, provided schemes are truly independent, shaped by and involving people using services, and completely honest about allowing clients to challenge all aspects of the services provided. Such schemes can also, within the obvious legal constraints, allow clients to shape key aspects of service. Policies on self-harm, seclusion, restraint, care planning and other issues can all be subject to appropriate client involvement.

The real challenge to managers of forensic services will be in ensuring that staff are adequately prepared and trained for this aspect of the *NHS Plan*. Advocacy schemes that leave staff defensive, bewildered or under threat are not good for anyone, least of all people using services. Sound investment in preparing staff and clients will pay off in the longer term.

A real issue in forensic services comes from the fact that many beds in this sector are provided outside the NHS. Technically, the *NHS Plan* does not apply to these settings. Over time, I am sure that independent sector providers catering for NHS patients will be required to meet *NHS Plan* targets via their contracts. Wise providers in this sector will not wait for NHS contracts to catch up with the ideas around advocacy, they will aim to meet these standards immediately. Another safeguard that can be provided by genuine independence is the scrutiny of complaints. The NHS system allows for some external review, but is this enough? Independent sector providers who are concerned with good practice have complaints systems which mirror those of the NHS. Real scrutiny of such information from someone outside the organisation can contribute to patient empowerment.

Increasingly throughout the UK, people who have experienced using services are setting up their own networks and many are becoming expert trainers. There are many examples of increased service user consultation and training, and smart organisations will keep a good database of such networks. In supporting self-advocacy, training staff and service planning, input from an able external consultant who has used services can be a rich source of development.

In October 2000, the Government accepted into law conventions from Europe involving human rights (House of Commons, 1998). This has profound implications for all that use forensic services and staff working within them, particularly around the issue of dangerous and severe personality disorder. As I write, Government is considering new plans to deal with this group of people (DoH, 1999). The professions in mental health have struggled for clarity around diagnosis and treatment in this area for decades. Yet Government are in danger of creating more muddle, with a misguided new label of 'severe and dangerous'. What clear meaning does this new definition actually convey?

The Government solution is to implement a new service, where such people can be confined, without limit of time, if they are assessed as being a societal risk. Where such an individual has already committed a serious offence and risk is self-evident, one can see the sense of the state wanting to continue detention. But here there must be robust legal and ethical scrutiny for individuals detained. What is more worrying is the idea suggested by Government that people who have committed no offence, but are labelled 'dangerous and severely personality disordered', might also be detained without limit of time.

The House of Commons Health Select Committee report into mental health raises fundamental questions about these issues and remains concerned that such proposals will leave the UK Government vulnerable to challenge under new human rights legislation (DoH, 2000a). Where might this leave staff working in such a system? The factor, which allows the building of trust and security through a therapeutic contract, is hope. People detained in forensic settings, regardless of diagnosis or legal status, hope that they will have a chance to rebuild their lives and move on to some framework of citizenship. That may, and sometimes does, take many years. But it is this that binds the healthy therapeutic balance in daily care.

If we are to detain people with difficult and challenging behaviours in this new service, where no certainty about potential for release is to be had, the implications for staff are frankly dangerous. If a group of individuals who have already committed murder in complex circumstances are detained, knowing there is little hope of moving on, what is to stop them murdering again? This alone would place staff and others in such environments at considerable risk. Where would staff be left in the inevitable legal challenges that would undoubtedly flow from this ill-conceived policy? In effect, we are creating a prison regime, but dressing it up under a health banner. If Government want this change, it would be wiser to implement it under the criminal justice system, not confuse the health system. The challenges of this strand of policy will need much reflection by those charged with the planning, management and delivery of forensic mental health services.

The final contemporary challenge for those in leadership roles must lie in how we recruit, retain, motivate and develop staff of the highest calibre for such services. We know that there is a problem in forensic services, with high vacancy rates in nursing, psychiatry and allied professions. As new monies are committed to the NHS under the *NHS Plan*, it will be crucial that leaders ensure that appropriate resources for education and staff development are considered in education consortia.

Our universities and other education providers need to understand the requirements of forensic mental health services.

There is a risk that education consortia debates will be dominated by the agendas of acute general hospitals. It is imperative that leaders develop clear strategies that influence the numbers entering mental health training and that the specialty gets sufficient attention in the allocation of resources to support quality post-graduate opportunities. These two factors will do much to influence issues around skill shortages in the workforce.

Research and development (R and D) opportunities in the specialty are too limited. If we are to attract and keep the best staff, we must ensure an expanded range of research and development activity. Professionals of quality in all disciplines are increasingly expecting research opportunities as part of their employment experience. Adequate resources in this neglected area will not happen by chance. Leaders must create the space for such activity and ensure sufficient resourcing. This is a key element of successful workforce planning and will become increasingly so.

Finally, new NHS developments will need to be reflected in the independent sector, where many forensic mental health beds are now provided. In the NHS, we are witnessing the development of new clinical career paths, with the development of new consultant grades in nursing and the professions allied to medicine. The best independent providers have been adept at supporting practice development and advanced clinical roles. In future, all independent providers will need to do so. Leaders in this sector should be tracking the use and development of these new consultant roles and ensuring that they are adapted and utilised effectively outside the NHS.

Key points

❊ Inhumane, institutionalised approaches and ill treatment in a large psychiatric hospital, where the author worked in the early nineteen seventies, led to complaints by junior staff and students and a regional inquiry. Later in his career, the author discovered other instances of very serious patient neglect, abuse and ill treatment in the UK and other European countries. However, student nurses and staff who 'whistle-blow' in response have faced considerable difficulties.

❊ Mental health service users' experiences are often ignored by statutory agencies and professionals. The treatment of minority group patients in most secure settings is cause for concern. Abuse of mental health service users is associated with staff's perception of them as 'different' or 'apart' from themselves. Individuals with mental health problems are marginalised and excluded in wider society, similar to processes in Nazi Germany.

❊ Secure services need to ensure a balance between 'security and public safety' and the provision of a 'therapeutic regime', with clear values which are not compromised. Problems in high secure hospitals relate to confusion about values; and conflicts between therapeutic goals and central Government policies requiring subjection to 'prison-like values and associated cultures'.

❊ Advocacy services in high secure hospitals must result in real empowerment, concerned with issues such as abuse and 'rights to information about treatment options.' Such schemes must be independent, with service user participation. The latter should include opportunities to question all aspects of service provision, and to contribute to policies and other important areas.

❊ The independent sector should have similar advocacy and complaints systems, and staff career pathways, to those in the NHS.

⌘ Government documents on 'dangerous people with severe personality disorder' have proposed that individuals who have not offended may be detained indefinitely. Such proposals are likely to be challenged under the Human Rights Act, 1998. They will leave individuals concerned without hope for the future, and place staff caring for them at risk.

⌘ Leaders of forensic services face challenges in relation to recruitment and retention (eg. in relation to research opportunities); and the motivation, development and education of staff. External consultants with service user experience can usefully inform 'self-advocacy, training staff and service planning'.

References

Beardshaw V (1981) *Conscientious Objectors at Work*. Social Audit, London

Department of Health (1999) *Report of the Committee of Inquiry into the Personality Disorder Unit*. Ashworth Special Hospital, HMSO, London

Department of Health (2000a) *Provision of NHS Mental Health Services, Volume 1*. Health Committee, The House of Commons, HMSO, London: July

Department of Health (2000b) *Report of a Review of Security in High Secure Hospitals* (The Tilt Report). DoH, London: May

Department of Health (2000c) *The NHS Plan*. Department of Health, London: July

Health Advisory Service (1986) *Report of the Health Advisory Service on Mental Health Services in West Lambeth DHA*. HAS, London

House of Commons (1998) Human Rights Act 1998, Chapter 42. The Stationery Office, London

House of Commons (2000) Health Committee Provision of Mental Health Services. Volume 1. HMSO, London

Rowden R (1981) Off the record, from one RMN to three others. *Nurs Mirror*, Sept 2, London

Sayce L (2000) *From Psychiatric Patient to Citizen. Overcoming Discrimination and Social Exclusion*. Macmillan, Basingstoke

South East Thames Regional Health Authority (1974) *Report of the Committee of Inquiry into St.Augustine's Hospital*. SE Thames RHA, London

12

Creating and maintaining strategies for empowering clients within high secure hospital settings

Lawrence Whyte and Gerry Carton

Introduction

The concept of empowerment has become increasingly important in discussions over the nature of contemporary healthcare practice (Gilbert, 1995). The emerging philosophical basis for health care is concerned itself with enabling individuals to achieve and maintain optimal physical, psychological and social well-being. One of the clinical areas where the empowerment philosophy might have difficulties in being realised is within high secure care. Part of the difficulties occurring may be to do with the nature of high secure hospitals themselves.

This chapter will focus upon attempts within high secure hospitals to create and maintain empowerment for clients. Central to any discussion of empowerment is its relationship with power itself. This requires that the effects of power within different locations or by different individual professions are identified and that the forms of social and clinical practice it produces are made explicit. The very nature of power in high secure hospitals makes them potentially disempowering institutions. Encouraging collaboration, co-operation, partnership and participation between those who reside, and those who work in these hospitals, produces tensions that need to be explored.

This chapter is divided into three discrete but inter-related sections. The first section deals with the nature of high secure hospital care within England and Wales. The second examines some of the tensions and problems of encouraging and fostering empowerment philosophies within these settings. The final section highlights some of the methods that have been employed within high secure hospitals to attempt to create and maintain client participation, collaboration between clients and staff and the desire for partnerships to emerge.

High secure hospitals — background

The nature of high secure hospital settings is arguably unique. Frequently referred to as 'special hospitals', they have often been cited as institutions where abuses of power have been evident, either through staff disempowerment of clients or clients' empowerment over staff (Boynton, 1980; Blom-Cooper, 1992; Fallon *et al*, 1999).

There are three high secure hospitals serving England and Wales: Ashworth, Broadmoor and Rampton. There is also the state hospital of Carstairs which serves Scotland and Northern Ireland. The majority of clients are referred from the courts and remand centres or from local psychiatric medium or low secure facilities, because they have become too difficult to manage. There are also serving prisoners who have been transferred to high secure hospital care under the conditions of the Mental Health Act 1983. Within the National Health Service Act 1977, the high secure hospitals are described as existing for the purpose of treating mentally disordered patients under conditions of special security on account of their dangerous, violent or criminal propensities. Such a purpose requires each of the three hospitals to combine three major functions:

❖ They are custodial institutions that aim to prevent individuals from engaging in acts that could be harmful to themselves or others.

❖ They are protective organisations seeking to safeguard the rights of clients detained under the Mental Health Act 1983.

❖ They are therapeutic hospitals whose purpose is to provide treatment that will enable clients to improve their health status and prepare them to return to less secure environments, or to the outside community, as soon as possible.

As institutions providing these three functions, the high secure hospitals are unique. However, they are also located within a network of other less secure psychiatric and learning disabilities facilities with which they supposedly interact. There has been considerable effort to improve the integration of high security hospitals with other agencies, institutions and secure organisations that could provide a full spectrum of care. The 'integrated system' for secure provision is often perceived as a pyramid. There are relatively small numbers of service users at the high secure pinnacle of the pyramid, fanning out into the much broader set of community-based services which, it is suggested, will need to be in place, both to prevent the need to move to high security and to enable people to move back into their own communities (Office for Public Management, 1999). *Figure 12.1* illustrates this pyramid structure.

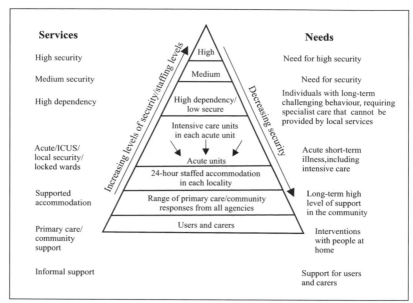

Figure 12.1: The needs-related pyramid of service provision

To be considered eligible for admission to a high security hospital, two criteria must be met. Firstly, the person must exhibit a mental disorder requiring compulsory treatment. Secondly, he or she must present a risk of being dangerous, violent or having criminal propensities. Given these criteria and the three functions of the high secure hospitals (custodial, protective and therapeutic) there is little doubt that there may be tensions around issues such as rights, responsibilities and privileges for those who reside or work within them.

High security hospitals are hybrid organisations in a number of ways. For example, on the one hand they present with many of the characteristics of the modern hospital (Matcha, 2000), on the other hand, the admission, discharge and length of stay statistics are relatively out of keeping with other mainstream mental health services (Special Hospitals Service Authority, 1995). Admissions to high secure hospitals are relatively low, as is discharge. Length of stay is long, approximately eight years on average. The client population within high security settings is relatively stable and unchanging.

In addition, the high secure hospital gives the impression of a prison environment, with features such as maximum high security perimeter fencing, surveillance monitoring through close circuit television and locked doors. However, greater freedom of movement is encouraged within the hospital's secure areas. Twenty-four-hour therapeutic services are offered, with the encouragement of client choice and autonomy, as part of the health model that is adopted.

The duality of roles of many clients is also a hybrid feature. As authors such as Adshead (1993, 1994) have argued, clients may be both perpetrators of criminal activities and violence, as well as being victims themselves of physical and sexual abuse (Bland *et al*, 1999). They are both dangerous and vulnerable. This is compounded by the social roles that staff have to engage in during their everyday encounters with these clients. As organisations, the high secure hospitals are managed as part of the National Health Service, yet provide services on behalf of the criminal justice system. While they have an emphasis upon the assessment, care and treatment of individuals with a mental illness and/or learning disability, they are also charged with the maintenance of public safety. Hence, the criteria for admission and discharge of clients is not solely determined by progression from illness to wellness but to other socially constructed criteria, such as risk and dangerousness.

Neither is the clinical profile straightforward. The client group of high security hospitals remains relatively constant. In November 1998, there was a total population of 1,335 clients. Approximately 87% (n=1,166) of the total population were male, with the remaining 13% (n=169) female (Fallon *et al*, 1999). This population of clients has been perceived as having quite diverse clinical needs (Special Hospitals Service Authority, 1995). There has been some concern, from a variety of studies, that a significant proportion of the client group is inappropriately placed. Estimates range from 20% to 45% of the total population (Office for Public Management, 1999). But Coid and Kahtan (2000) suggest caution about such estimates. Through an analysis of client admissions to high security hospitals over a six-year period, they found that there was little evidence to suggest that lower levels of secure provision, such as medium secure units, reduced the demand for beds in high secure hospitals. Admissions to high security hospitals were characterised by more serious behavioural disturbances and more serious offences, the clients had more extensive previous criminal histories and were more likely to have primary and co-morbid diagnosis of personality disorder and diagnoses associated with sexual offending (Coid and Kahtan, 2000).

Clients categorised as suffering from mental illness, under the Mental Health Act 1983, form the largest group within the total population, accounting for about two thirds of clients. Many of these clients are likely to suffer from more than one clinical syndrome or illness, giving a complex profile that might be further influenced by additional developmental disorders, physical disorders, histories of substance abuse and patterns of offending that are usually of a serious nature (Special Hospitals Service Authority, 1995). Clients detained under the legal classification of psychopathic disorder alone comprise about 25% of the high secure hospital population and a further 11% of clients have the legal classification of psychopathic disorder with another classification (Fallon *et al*, 1999). Again, there is a heterogeneous mixture of clinical characteristics, with considerable diversity in clinical and behavioural complexity. While the majority of clients are male, the emerging literature on the constellation of clinical problems surrounding women clients with personality disorders suggests different problems and different needs (Hemingway, 1996; Liebling, Chipchase and Velangi, 1997; Lart, 1999). It has long been recognised that clients from ethnic minority origins are disproportionately over-represented in high security services (Kaye and Lingiah, 2000; Special Hospitals Service Authority, 1995).

The hybrid nature of high security hospitals, and the complex and diverse needs of the client group may create tension and uncertainty among staff. It is suggested that nursing staff, in particular, who are in most frequent contact with clients, experience tension between the two conflicting roles of custodian and therapist (Burrow, 1991, 1993; Whyte, 1985). As suggested earlier, the client group may be perceived as occupants of a number of roles themselves, such as; patient, detainee, perpetrator and victim.

Each of these roles carries with it certain expectations and behaviours. *Figure 12.2* outlines some of these. Clearly, both staff and clients are expected to manage at least two roles that may be competing and potentially conflicting in their relationships with each other. While the relationships between some of the roles might be mutually complementary (eg. therapist-patient, custodian-detainee), the potential for role ambiguity and role conflict may manifest itself when mutually incompatible roles are enacted (eg. therapist-detainee, custodian-victim).

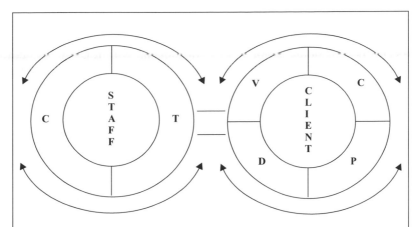

C = Custodian
- ensures public safety
- security as primary objective
- ensures compliance to rules and procedures
- restricts movement
- surveillance and monitoring

C = Client
- motivated to get better
- accepts illness state
- trusting
- seeks empowerment
- ownership of participation
- willingness to disclose
- expresses remorse

T = Therapist
- offers hope and path to wellness
- openness, acceptance
- encouragement of partnership
- development of mutual trust
- accepts illness state

D = Detainee
- potentially dangerous
- a rival
- compliant to rules and procedures
- a security risk

V = Victim
- passive
- protectionist
- emotionally affected
- angry
- revengeful

P = Perpetrator
- predatory
- opportunist
- active
- aggressive
- risk of recidivism

Figure 12.2: Roles and expectations of clients and staff within high secure hospitals

Role ambiguity may occur for either of the actors, client or staff, if there is little information available on what the expected performance should be or if the participants within a role system disagree on the role expectations for a particular role. For example, a nurse who acts as a therapist for a patient may have emotional difficulties in knowing how to adopt a custodial role. Collins (2000) suggests that this may be problematic for newly qualified nurses entering secure environments, who may have limited experience of security duties. Similarly, a client transferred from a prison to a high security hospital may have difficulty in perceiving nurses as therapists if his/her previous experience suggests that they act mainly as warders.

Role conflict is the process whereby the person enacting the set of roles expected of them, perceives existing role expectations as being contradictory or mutually exclusive. This occurs when the role occupant has difficulty fulfilling role obligations (expectations and demand for a role occupant) because the expectations themselves are contradictory. A number of authors have suggested this potential for role conflicts between the roles of custodian and therapist within a secure environment (Burrow, 1993; Liou, 1995) or within the creation of a therapeutic relationship (Sullivan, 1998; McGuire, 1997). Surprisingly, there is little available research on the potential role ambiguity or role conflicts that clients might experience through being on the receiving end of therapy, as detained individuals or as perpetrators and/or victims.

It can be concluded that the creation and maintenance of empowerment for clients within high secure hospital settings is influenced by a number of factors. These include: the relatively stable populations of high secure hospitals, the complexity of clinical, behavioural and developmental conditions of these populations, ambiguity of the roles of high secure hospitals themselves and the resulting uncertainty that this ambiguity creates for the main actors within that setting, ie. professional healthcare staff and clients. A further factor is isolation.

Martin with Evans (1984), in a critique of the failure of care in large psychiatric and learning disabilities hospitals, identified six types of isolation that may have been contributory to the poor care and management of clients within these institutions. These were:

❖ Geographical isolation: Most of the institutions were situated outside main urban centres.

❖ Immediate isolation: Certain wards within the same hospital were isolated from each other and operated as semi-autonomous units.

❖ Personal isolation: Individuals were left in charge of large numbers of difficult-to-manage clients.

❖ Consultant isolation: Certain wards and departments were rarely visited by their responsible medical officers.

❖ Intellectual isolation: The absence of professional stimulus, training and education opportunities.

❖ Private isolation: Those clients who were subject to abuse were least likely to be regularly visited by relatives.

These identified factors suggest that the everyday encounters between clients and staff within high security hospitals are complex and dynamic. They are also subject to changes in policy directives at a national level. For example, the enquiry into allegations of abuse at Ashworth Hospital headed by Blom-Cooper (1992) advocated a stronger emphasis upon therapeutic imperatives, with some liberalisation of practices that would empower patients and challenge staff to examine their predominantly security-orientated models of care. By the time of the Fallon enquiry (1999) at the same hospital, some of these practices, albeit misinterpreted, were seen as critical indicators of a breakdown in security measures, resulting in a re-emphasis upon the primacy of the protection of the public and the maintenance of high levels of security.

The constantly changing perceptions of how high secure hospitals should be operated, the cluster of isolation factors, the stable client and staff populations, the complexity of the behaviours and diagnosis of the client group and the limited development of 'medical technology' to influence severe clinical and behavioural conditions, all contribute to the sense of ambiguity and uncertainty that emerges between staff and clients through their interactions. A clear example of this is given in the discussion about 'rights' and 'privileges' that the Fallon report (1999) posited.

While basically endorsing the earlier Blom-Cooper inquiry team's report that gave clients a much stronger voice, Fallon was critical of ways in which the liberalisation ethos of Blom-Cooper was re-interpreted by staff and clients within Ashworth Hospital, and particularly within the unit dealing with individuals with the legal classification of psychopathic disorder. Fallon (1999) draws attention to the need for staff and clients to understand the distinction between a person's rights and privileges within a high security setting.

Fallon (1999) argues that the failure by staff and clients to understand these distinctions was a fundamental pre-requisite for the events that occurred. In particular, staff felt unable to challenge or implement certain security and therapeutic practices because of fears and anxieties of being perceived as invading clients' rights. As Fallon (1999) argues:

> *There is a distinction first of all between fundamental human rights and other rights people enjoy as members of particular nations or groups within them. The main difference is that fundamental human rights should be considered immutable. Social rights are not immutable and they are closely associated with duties. For example, people living in a country have a duty to comply with the laws of that country and if they breach those laws they can be punished and also lose rights.*

(Fallon, 1999, p. 91)

This argument continues to suggest that a sentence of imprisonment involves the loss of the rights to freedom for the duration of a sentence; and that while resident within an institution, people should abide by its rules which are geared towards the promotion of the welfare and well being of others with whom they live and are in close everyday contact.

While there may be clarity concerning the rights and privileges of prisoners, this is less clear in relation to clients in high security hospitals. Certain groups of the latter, particularly those with the legal classification of 'psychopathic disorder', will exploit and redefine these distinctions if the clarity is blurred. In the situation described in the Fallon Inquiry, staff, and consequently, clients, perceived 'privileges' to be 'rights'.

Given the uncertainty and ambiguity about the extent to which clients were allowed to, or could earn 'privileges', and the unclear boundaries between 'rights' and 'privileges', operating within such a closed and isolated institution, staff and clients could be seen to act in different ways. Clients with personality disorders, who are generally articulate, intelligent and creative, have the opportunity to challenge and manipulate the interpretation of the blurred boundaries, and exploit the uncertainty and ambiguity experienced by staff. On the other hand, staff, confronted by very articulate individuals who are difficult to control, retreat away from confrontation, thereby surrendering greater control to the clients.

Menzies (1970) suggests that some health professionals, such as nurses, cope with the demanding and less rewarding aspects of their work by adopting defensive strategies that help them to externalise, rather than internalise, these work pressures. Under difficult and threatening work conditions, these socially constructed defence mechanisms enable healthcare workers to manage their fears and anxieties about this work. Menzies (1960, 1970) described various social defence mechanisms used by nurses in these situations. These include a distribution of tasks in order to 'split up the nurse-patient relationship' (Menzies, 1960, p. 101), so that the potential for developing this therapeutically becomes minimised. Other defence mechanisms include a depersonalisation process, where the unique significance of the individual client's experience is denied. There may also be a reliance upon rituals and task performance and the meeting of the needs of a 'batch' of clients, rather than those related to specific individuals. Another mechanism consists of eliminating the need to make decisions and reducing the weight of responsibility in decision making.

Strategies employed to maintain and enhance empowerment for clients within high secure hospital settings

Given the inherent tensions and difficulties involved, multiple and wide-ranging strategies are needed to develop a balance between clients' universal rights, treatment rights and entitlement of privileges. For the purposes of clarity, the strategies that might be useful in high security hospital settings have been categorised under four main headings: personal qualities and attitudes, professional strategies, organisational strategies and external strategies. Each of these will be discussed. *Figure 12.3* outlines these in diagrammatic form.

Personal qualities and attributes of staff

As Onyett (1992) points out, very few people seek help from mental health services with enthusiasm. The qualities and attributes of staff within these services might be helped by guidelines for engagement with clients. The latter should aim to maximise the chances of achieving a good solid foundation on which to base a helpful relationship, while simultaneously ensuring that the autonomy and rights of clients are not infringed. Onyett's (1992) guidelines for engagement include: being prepared, attending to issues of difference, making yourself a real person who comes from somewhere, getting alongside the client, showing respect, establishing links with individuals known and trusted by the client, persisting where appropriate and being flexible enough to try something different. Having established the foundations of a positive relationship through engagement, Onyett suggests that the focus should change to one of developing an effective relationship with the client for collaborative working. This should be guided by; being clear about what you can and cannot do, leaving clients with as much power as possible, giving permission for the client to rely on you and communicating effectively.

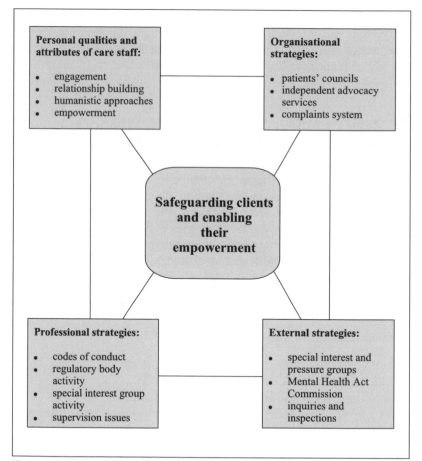

Figure 12.3: An outline of some of the strategies that seek to safeguard and enhance clients' rights

These generally humanistic guidelines are supported by other authors. Read and Wallcraft (1992) recommend that staff should adhere to the following criteria when trying to empower clients:

- letting the client know their rights
- asking them what they want from the service
- recognising the client's strengths, capabilities, potential and talents
- talking and listening to clients and giving as much information as they can assimilate about their treatment, management and the options open to them.

From a psychologist's perspective, Strasburger *et al* (1997) suggest the development of a therapeutic alliance in which the helper attempts to ally with that part of the client that is seeking to change, to give up psychopathological symptoms and to resume or develop healthy adaptations. However, the skills of empathy, therapeutic neutrality and anonymity (which aid the development and interpretation of transference and the mobilisation of clinically useful projections onto the therapist) are clearly compromised by the legal processes involved in care.

Jackson and Stevenson (2000) found that there were a number of nursing strategies that needed to be developed which could maximise client autonomy and well-being. These include the mental health nurse's visibility and accessibility to clients; and ability to move across domains of language, in order to act as interpreter to fellow professionals. Other factors include the relatively high level of contact between nurses and patients; and the opportunity to develop the form and function of clinical supervision in support of the nurse's role.

Professional strategies

In addition to being an individual practitioner in his/her own right, each health professional's practice, and the extent to which (s)he can empower clients, is controlled by a professional body, with specific regulatory functions and a code of conduct.

Regulatory body activity

To reflect the responsibility vested in them by clients and by society, healthcare professionals have a professional obligation or duty to account for their actions (including those intended to facilitate client empowerment). Professionals have accountability not only to clients and the public, but also to the law, their peers and managers and to the appropriate regulatory body. The latter includes the General Medical Council (GMC) and the Nursing and Midwifery Council (NMC) which, in April 2002, replaced the United Kingdom Central Council for Nursing, Midwifery and Health Visiting (UKCC).

Professional regulatory bodies protect the interests of clients, including those in high security hospitals, as well as the general public. According to Pyne (1998), this is achieved through five key elements. These include the maintenance of a professional register, which details the registered practitioners in a particular profession. Mechanisms controlling entry to the register also protect client and public interests. Such mechanisms include the regulation of appropriate education and training in an approved institution, at the end of which an individual has demonstrated possession of the appropriate knowledge and skills that make him/her eligible to embark on a career as a professional practitioner. Pyne also considers mechanisms to ensure removal of the authority to practice. Regulatory bodies have powers and procedures whereby, in the interests of clients and the public, they can remove or suspend a person's registration and prevent him/her from practising as a professional. Regulatory bodies also develop strategies to maintain fitness for purpose, enabling practitioners to develop professionally and base their work (including the facilitation of client empowerment and participation) on current best practice.

Professional codes of conduct

In addition, regulatory bodies expect their registrants to adhere to codes of conduct intended to protect clients and the public. Such codes are concerned with the moral dimensions of health care. According to Downie and Calman (1994), codes are important because they state some of the principles intended to underlie professional activity. In addition, they indicate some consensus on how professional activity should or should not be conducted at the basic principle level.

The *Code of Professional Conduct* of the NMC requires nurses and midwives to, 'promote the interests of patients and clients' (NMC, 2002, p. 4, Clause 2.4). Commenting on a similar statement in Clause 1 of the former UKCC's *Professional Code of Conduct*, Furlong (1999) states that it:

> ... *addresses the power balance, and power imbalance, of [professional – client] relationships. It identifies that*

*nurses, midwives and health visitors are perfectly placed
to provide support to their patients and in doing so, it is
asserted... will be able to ensure that patients will be able to
participate fully in any decisions concerning their health
care. Implicit in Clause 1 is the registered practitioner's
role as patient advocate.*

*... Patients or clients are unable to make informed choices
until they are empowered...*

(Furlong, 1999, p. 17)

Codes of conduct have several limitations. They delineate the ethical principles by which professionals are expected to abide, although it is a truism that individuals bring their own personal values to their professional lives. Mercer *et al* (1999) outline research which found that, in one high secure hospital, there was a tension between nurses' professional and personal values. The latter were rooted in those of wider society, which construed certain patients as being 'evil'.

Codes of conduct tend to be unidisciplinary, rather than multidisciplinary. In addition, there are aspects of health care that are not necessarily expressed through codes, eg. the cultivation of certain attitudes, such as compassion or the instilling of hope, which are not reducible to rules.

Special interest activity

Professional associations, such as the Royal College of Psychiatrists and the Royal College of Nursing have special interest groups and forums that seek to disseminate 'best' practice (including client empowerment and participation) to individual practitioners. These offer the opportunity for members to influence the knowledge and skills base for their profession within a specified speciality, such as forensic health care.

Professionals, therefore, have a range of mechanisms by which they can seek to maximise the interests of their own professional group as well as improve the care of clients. The influences of professional strategies have been growing within high secure hospitals over the past decade.

Organisational strategies

As well as individual and professional body influences, each of the high security hospitals has developed organisational strategies to maximise clients' autonomy and ensure the balance between individuals' rights and privileges, while maintaining public safety. Three main organisational mechanisms exist. These are patients' councils, independent advocacy services and complaints systems.

Patients' councils

In high secure hospitals, it is often difficult for the people being cared for to get their voice heard. This might magnify their feelings of powerlessness and they may feel fearful of the consequences of complaining or lack effective channels to express their views about the services received. A patients' council provides a formal mechanism through which the hospital management and other professional groups can consult with and respond to, matters raised by clients. The aim of the council is for people to have a collective say in the improvement of care, treatment and quality of life during their time in hospital.

Each of the high security hospitals has its own patients' council which usually comprise elected or self-appointed client representatives, who meet on a regular basis and bring concerns to the attention of the hospital management. As Curran and Grimshaw (1996) suggest, the advantages of patients' councils include the fostering of empowerment, improved understanding of clients' needs and concerns; and enabling the smoother running of the hospital by encouraging staff and clients to work together.

Independent advocacy services

Each of the high secure hospitals has external contracts with specified mental health agencies to provide independent advocacy services for its clients. Independent advocacy is important for two reasons according to Wetherell (2000). Firstly, putting the responsibility on healthcare staff to provide advocacy may place individuals in positions of compromise as they try to balance conflicts of interest, in terms of their professional and personal values. In addition, independent advocacy is likely to be more effective in ensuring that vulnerable individuals in care have their rights and needs heard.

Complaints system

The high secure hospitals have established a complaints process that complies with National Health Service procedure, as defined in the document *Acting on Complaints* published in March, 1995 and supplemented by National Health Service's *Guidance on the Implementation of the New Complaints Procedure* (National Health Service Executive, 1996). These hospitals apply all elements of the

NHS guidance without exception. The system is designed to be used as part of a quality improvement process.

In one high secure hospital, any complaints involving alleged offences by patients or staff are automatically referred to an independent investigation by the local police service. This situation has emerged as a consequence of an earlier police investigation into that hospital, and enables patients to have ready access to the police in order to pursue such complaints.

Compared with complaints received by other mental health service providers, in high secure hospitals, complaints broadly relate to interpersonal relationships, with a focus upon violence. In other mental health services, complaints are more likely to concern processes of care: for instance, cancelled appointments, waiting times, changes in medical staff or lack of opportunity to meet with the named nurse.

This contrast is interesting and a number of possible explanations can be offered. One such explanation may be patients' perceived lack of control within high secure hospitals. In relation to their rights to comment on processes of care, patients may be concerned that complaints in this area may adversely affect their status as detained patients, the lessening of restrictions and their eventual discharge. This may or may not be the case, but it does highlight a potential limitation of utilising a complaints procedure as the only safeguard for patients in high secure hospitals. Such a system needs to be one of a battery of arrangements to overcome this particular conflict of power and control to ensure that user empowerment is real within these facilities.

External strategies

As well as the mechanisms for individual practitioners, professional activities and organisational strategies that seek to maintain the balance between meeting clients' rights and privileges and ensuring public safety, there are a number of external mechanisms that exist. Three of these will be described: special interest and pressure groups, the Mental Health Act Commission and inquiries and inspections.

Special interest and pressure groups

Earlier in this chapter, it was argued that the population of high secure hospitals was heterogeneous in its needs and demands. There are, therefore, several special interest and pressure groups, external to the hospitals, that seek to ensure that the specific needs of particular client groups are met. Specific aims of WISH (Women in secure hospitals), outlined in their Annual Report, 1999 to 2000, are given in the box below.

**Aims and objectives of WISH
(Women in secure hospitals)**

'To promote equality of opportunity and respond to the individual needs of women during, after and at risk of secure psychiatric containment.'
'To be accessible to women who are at risk of secure psychiatric containment and work to prevent inappropriate admissions.'
'To inform, advise and give voice to women in secure psychiatric settings and reduce their isolation.'
'To work constructively with staff and managers to improve the quality and appropriateness of care for women in secure psychiatric settings.'
'To empower and support women on discharge from secure psychiatric settings.'
'To promote provision of appropriate resources and facilities within the community.'
'To influence the appropriate reform of secure mental health provision for women, in tandem with the statutory and voluntary sector, by raising awareness, initiating research and promoting sound therapeutic strategies.'

From WISH, undated
Glimmers of Hope. The WISH Annual Report, 1999–2000, p. 4

Through their aims, pressure groups such as WISH have been influential in putting the needs of their clients high on the agenda of health service and secure hospital managers, and in raising awareness of their special needs.

The Mental Health Act Commission

The 1983 Mental Health Act gave the Mental Health Act Commission responsibility for keeping under review the implementation of the powers and duties conferred by the Act, as they relate to detained clients. All those admitted to high secure hospitals are detained under the Act and come under the Commission's remit. In order to fulfil its remit, the Commission has rights of access to all detained clients at any reasonable time and the right to interview them in private. It also has rights of access to documentation relating to their detention.

Inquiries and inspections

Organisations such as the high secure hospitals can expect close scrutiny from a number of organisations. Kaye and Franey (1998) distinguish between inspections and inquiries. Inspections include regular reviews of the high secure hospitals by independent established bodies, which evaluate the implementation of specific aspects of care, treatment and security. Kaye and Franey list over fifteen bodies that may carry out periodic inspections. Inquiries are concerned with the appointment of an individual or a team to review the significance of an incident or series of incidents, usually where it is thought that something has gone wrong. Examples of such inquiries are; Fallon *et al* (1999), Blom-Cooper (1992) and Boynton (1980).

Inspections and inquiries seek to offer reassurance to clients, their relatives, staff and the general public about what goes on behind the doors of a relatively closed institution. Martin with Evans (1984), set out four criteria for inquiries to be successful. They should: allay public alarm, discover the facts and pass judgement on what took place, provide an adequate explanation of what has happened and, in the longer term, provide a good basis for developing higher standards of care.

Conclusion

This chapter has sought to summarise three discrete yet related issues. Firstly, the nature of high security hospitals was examined and in particular, the diverse needs and demands of a complex and varied population of clients were highlighted. Secondly, some of the possible tensions and problems associated with trying to encourage and foster empowerment philosophies within these settings were discussed. Finally, there was a review of the strategies and mechanisms to ensure the balance between clients' rights, privileges, safety of the public and prevention of abuse.

These issues are not exhaustive. The history of the high secure hospitals would suggest that, despite the existence of these varied and diverse mechanisms, there is enormous difficulty in establishing and maintaining this balance. All three of the high secure hospitals have been the subject of damning external enquiries over the past two decades. Consistently, prominent voices have argued for their closure (Bluglass, 1992; Fallon *et al*, 1999). In many ways, despite their opening up to the wider NHS, the high secure hospitals remain relatively isolated, geographically and professionally. Whether the strategies created and maintained to foster empowerment within these hybrid organisations are sufficient, only the advent of the next scandal (or otherwise) will tell.

Key points

❋ Abuses of power in high secure hospitals have been cited. These organisations are unique in their combined aims of public protection, safeguarding patients' rights and providing treatment. There can be tensions between these aims, reflected in aspects of a prison environment, but with therapeutic services.

❋ Many high secure clients have been victims, as well as perpetrators, of crime. While estimates suggest that a significant proportion is inappropriately placed, one study found that most clients, compared with those in medium secure units, had histories of more serious and extensive offending, and more complex mental health problems.

❋ Clients from minority ethnic groups are over-represented in high secure hospitals. The small minority of women patients have specific needs. There are relatively small numbers of clients in high secure, compared with medium and low secure services.

❋ Both clients and staff occupy multiple and potentially conflicting roles. There is a particular role conflict in staff roles of 'custodian' and 'therapist', and how these are perceived by clients.

❋ Client empowerment in high secure hospitals is influenced by 'relatively stable populations', the complexity of clients' problems, the hospitals' 'ambiguity of roles', and the uncertainty this causes clients and staff. Various types of isolation are also influential. Staff may use defensive strategies to manage difficulties encountered in their work.

⌘ Empowerment is also affected by changes in central Government policy. Thus, the Blom-Cooper Inquiry into Ashworth Hospital emphasised client empowerment. The Fallon Inquiry, published seven years later, criticised practices intended to empower as adversely affecting security and public protection; and distinguished between the rights and privileges of clients.

⌘ Aspects of staff-client relationships and communication can be empowering. These include 'development of a therapeutic alliance'; collaborative working; enabling clients to have power; information about patients' rights and other issues; recognition of patients' positive attributes; and accessibility. However, it has been argued that empowerment of mental health service users is 'compromised by... legal processes'.

⌘ The Nursing and Midwifery council influences empowerment through its regulatory functions, including those concerning professional accountability, registration, fitness to practice and the *Code of professional conduct*. Professional associations spread good practice related to empowerment and participation.

⌘ Organisational strategies influencing empowerment in high secure hospitals include patients' councils, independent advocacy services and complaints systems. These are concerned with patients' rights and needs, and the opportunity to be heard. A variety of organisational strategies is needed to overcome problems concerned with power and control.

References

Adshead G (1993) Victims and survivors. *Curr Opin Psychiatry* **6**: 758–63

Adshead G (1994) Damage: Trauma and violence in a sample of women referred in a forensic service. *Behav Sci Law* **12**: 235–49

Bland J, Mezey G, Dolan B (1999) Special women, special needs. A descriptive study of female special hospital patients. *J Forensic Psychiatry* **10**(1): 34–45

Bluglass R (1992) The special hospitals. *Br Med J* **305**: 323–4

Burrow S (1991) The special hospital nurse and the dilemma of therapeutic custody. *J Adv Nurs Health Care* **1**(3): 21–38

Burrow S (1993) An outline of the forensic nursing role. *Br J Nurs* **2**(18): 899–904

Coid J, Kahtan N (2000) Are special hospitals needed? *J Forensic Psychiatry* **11**(1): 17–35

Collins M (1999) The practitioner new to the role of forensic psychiatric nurse in the UK. In: Robinson D, Kettles A, eds. *Forensic Nursing and Multidisciplinary Care of the Mentally Disordered Offender*. Jessica Kingsley, London

Curran C, Grimshaw C (1996) Brief guide to making a patients'council work in a psychiatric hospital. *Open Mind* **80**: 28

Department of Health (1992) *Report of the Committee of Inquiry into Complaints about Ashworth Hospital*. (Authors: Blom-Cooper, Sir L, Brown M, Dolan K, Murphy E.) Cmnd 2028. HMSO, London

Department of Health (1995) *Acting on Complaints. The Government's Revised Policy and Proposals for a New NHS Complaints Procedure in England*. March, 1995. EL (95) 37

Department of Health (1999) *Making a Difference*. DoH, London

Department of Health (1999) *Report of the Committee of Inquiry into the Personality Disorder Unit, Ashworth Special Hospital,Volume 1*. (Authors: Fallon P, Bluglass R, Edwards B, Daniels G.) Cmnd 4194–11. The Stationery Office, London: January

Department of Health (1999) *Report of the Review of Rampton Hospital*. (Chair: Boynton, Sir J.) Cmnd 8073. HMSO, London

Department of Health (2001) *NHS Plan — An Action Guide for Nurses Midwives and Health Visitors*. DoH, London

Downie RS, Calman KC (1994) *Healthy Respect — Ethics in Health Care*. 2nd edn. Oxford Medical, Oxford

Furlong S (1999) Clause 1. Being there. In: Heywood Jones I, ed. *The UKCC Code of Conduct. A Critical Guide*. Nursing Times Books, London: chap 1

Gilbert T (1995) Nursing: Empowerment and the problem of power. *J Adv Nurs* **21**: 865–71

Hemingway C (1996) *Special Women? The Experience of Women in the Special Hospital System*. Avebury, Aldershot

Hogg C (1999) *Patients power and Politics. From patients to citizens*. Sage Publications, London

Jackson S, Stevenson C (2000) What do people need psychiatric and mental health nurses for? *J Adv Nurs* **31**(2): 378–88

Kaye C, Franey A, eds (1998) *Managing High Security Psychiatric Care*. Jessica Kinsgley, London

Kaye C, Lingiah T, eds (2000) *Race, Culture and Ethnicity in Secure Psychiatric Practice. Working with Difference*. Jessica Kingsley, London

Lart R, Payne K, Beaumont B, MacDonald G, Mistry T (1999) *Women and Secure Psychiatric Services: A Literature Review*. CRD. Report 14. NHS Centre for Reviews and Dissemination, University of York

Liebling H, Chipchase H, Velangi R (1997) Why do women harm themselves — surviving special hospitals. *Feminism and Psychology* **7**: 427–37

Liou KT (1995) Role stress and job stress among detention care workers. *Criminal Justice and Behaviour* **22**(4): 425–36

Martin J with Evans D (1984) *Hospitals in Trouble*. Robertson, Oxford

Matcha D (2000) *Medical Sociology*. Allyn and Bacon, Massachusetts

McGuire J (1997) Ethical dilemmas in forensic clinical psychology. *Legal and Criminological Psychol* **2**: 177–92

Menzies IEP (1960) A case study in the functioning of social systems as a defence against anxiety. *Hum Relations* **13**(2): 95–121

Menzies IEP (1970) *The Function of Social Systems as a Defence Against Anxiety — A Report of a Study on the Nursing Service of a General Hospital*. Tavistock Institute, London

Mercer D, Mason T, Richman J (1999) Good and evil in the crusade of care. Social constructions of mental disorders. *J Psychosoc Nurs Ment Health Serv* **37**(9): 13–17

National Health Service Executive (1996) *Complaints. Listening... Acting... Improving. Guidance on Implementation of the NHS Complaints Procedure*. Department of Health, London. EL (96) 19

Nursing and Midwifery Council (2002) *Code of Professional Conduct*. NMC, London

Office for Public Management (1999) *Secure Futures: High Security Psychiatric Services*. Office for Public Management, London

Onyett S (1992) *Case Management in Mental Health*. Chapman and Hall, London

Pyne R (1998) *Professional Discipline in Nursing, Midwifery and Health Visiting*. 3rd edn. Blackwell, Oxford

Read J, Wallcraft J (1992) *Guidelines for Empowering Users of Mental Health Services*. Confederation of Health Service Employees/MIND, London

Special Hospital Services Authority (1995) *Service Strategies for Secure Care*. SHSA, London

Strasburger L, Gutheil MD, Brockley A (1997) On wearing two hats: Role conflict in serving as both psychotherapist and expert witness. *Am J Psychiatry* **154**(4): 448–56

Sullivan P (1998) Therapeutic interactions and mental health nursing. *Nurs Standard* **12** (45): 39–42

United Kingdom Central Council for Nursing, Midwifery and Health Visiting (1992) *Code for Professional Conduct for the Nurse, Midwife and Health Visitor*. UKCC, London

Wetherell A (2000) Good advocacy: the vital ingredients. *Mental Health Practice* **3**(6): 9–11

Whyte L (1985) Safe as houses — custodial care or therapeutic interventions. *Nurs Mirror* **81**(23): 48

Women in Secure Hospitals (Undated) *Glimmers of Hope*. The WISH Annual Report, 1999–2000. WISH, London

13

Ethics committees, vulnerable groups and paternalism: the case for considering the benefits of participating in qualitative research interviews

John R Cutcliffe

Introduction

In one significant way, qualitative research studies are no different from quantitative studies, in that both **forms** of study present potential ethical issues which need to be considered. According to Lipson (1994), ethical issues in qualitative research are often less visible and more subtle than issues in survey or experimental research. Such differences are due to the inherent (emergent) nature (and design) of qualitative methods. It follows that if ethical issues in qualitative studies are more subtle, then they may require additional scrutiny in the hope that this leads to rigorous consideration and subsequent cogent arguments/positions.

The reader could be forgiven for wondering; what does ethical issues in qualitative research have to do with issues of empowerment? In response to this question, the central proposition of this chapter is that decisions made by ethical committees regarding the approval/disapproval of some qualitative research studies can have a direct impact on the empowerment of certain groups of people. In order to consider this proposition, the author will focus on the issue of over-paternalism by ethics committees with regard to vulnerable groups; in this instance, the vulnerable group of ex-clients who have received counselling.

The role of the local research ethics committee (LREC)

Without wishing to enter into a detailed examination of the history of LRECs, it is necessary to provide a synopsis which describes the rationale and function of these committees. Following key events in the development of research ethics, namely the Nuremberg trials and the Declaration of Helsinki (1964), the Royal College of Physicians recommended the introduction of ethics committees. Soon after this, the Department of Health stated that hospitals were to operate such committees. Since then, the Royal College of Physicians has continued to play a significant role in the debates over research ethics and produce guidelines for the operation of such committees (see Royal College of Physicians, 1990, 1996). The 1990 (p. 3) guidelines stated that the objectives of local research ethics committees (LRECs) would be to:

> ... *maintain ethical standards of practice in research, to protect subjects of research from harm, to preserve subjects' rights and to provide reassurance to the public that this is being done.*

Subsequent to this, the Department of Health (1991) issued recommendations for establishing LRECs and in 1994, guidelines for their operation. Consequently, LRECs comprised of eight to twelve members (from a wide variety of backgrounds) who have 'sound judgement and relevant experience' are appointed. This committee, which should include two lay committee members then have the remit of making decisions in relation to research which involves NHS patients (past and present), access to patient records or for research taking place on NHS premises. However, while carrying out their remit, LRECs are faced with resolving many ethical dilemmas and, according to Beauchamp and Childress (1994), one of the key dilemmas is that of paternalism; balancing the conflict between beneficence and autonomy.

Paternalism and ethics committees

Garritson and Davis (1983, p. 18) define paternalism as an action,

> ... *which restricts a person's liberty justified exclusively by consideration for that person's own good or welfare and carried out either against his present will or his prior commitment.*

According to Beauchamp and Childress (1994), the root meaning of paternalism is: the principle and practice of paternal administration; government as by a father; the claim or attempt to supply the needs or to regulate the life of a nation or community in the same way as a father does for his children. It is important to note that this paradigmatic form of justified paternalism starts with **incompetent children** in need of paternal supervision and extends to other **incompetents** in need of treatment analogous to beneficent paternal guidance (Beauchamp and Childress, 1994). If we consider the implications of this root meaning in the case of former counselling clients, the inference is that these people are similar (or the same?) as incompetent children or other incompetents.

Whether or not respect for the autonomy of patients should have priority over professional beneficence has become a central problem in biomedical ethics (Beauchamp and Childress, 1994). On the one hand, proponents of autonomy rights for patients point out that the principle of respect for autonomy indicates that a person has the right to make their own decisions. On the other hand, proponents of the physician's primary obligation being beneficence posit that the physician's primary obligation is the person's medical benefit, not to promote autonomous decision making (Beauchamp and Childress, 1994). Members of LRECs face the same ethical dilemma when considering research proposals. This bioethical discourse contains an implicit assumption that the medical profession claims 'ownership' of the person and some have noted the inherent paternalism of this approach (Cartwright, 1998). Since LRECs most often have a membership that includes a significant medical representation, it can be argued that the discourse of 'ownership' of people (patients) is replicated or reiterated within the LREC.

There is concern with the idea of an intermediary body such as ethics committees deciding on consent issues for a third party. Some of this concern appears to be grounded in the arguments for respecting the person's right to autonomy, and possibly that there is the potential for studies to be rejected by ethics committees because of what appears to be unsound design. In particular, concerns that an ethics committee would make the assumption that if interviewees consent to talking about difficult, traumatic, or emotionally ladened experiences, this may somehow cause the person harm. The interview somehow re-traumatises the interviewee and violates the obligation to do no harm. Such assumptions of ethics committees are maybe most noticeable when the study involves accessing vulnerable groups.

Vulnerable groups

Lasagna (1970) reasoned that vulnerable groups are captive populations, including; the mentally ill, the acutely ill, and the terminally ill. Usher and Holmes (1997) argue that vulnerable research participants are those that are considered to be unable or less able, to make autonomous decisions regarding their participation in research. McLeod (1996) argued that counselling is a sensitive topic for research since the process of counselling may sometimes be associated with great vulnerability in clients. Therefore, it can be seen that counselling clients are regarded as a further example of a vulnerable group, and if one accepts that position, that it is the sensitivity of the topic that indicates counselling clients as a vulnerable group, then perhaps the same could be said of ex-clients (ExCs), ie. clients who have completed their therapy.

According to Watson (1982), when considering whether or not people from these populations should be asked to participate in research studies there are several key factors to consider. The most frequently cited of these factors are; the seriousness and probability of risk to the patient, whether or not the subject or society receives any benefits, and the capability of the subject to give informed consent. As stated previously, the issue of risk to benefit ratio can be regarded as balancing the first two of these issues. However, different ethical theories/positions may produce different standpoints when considering risk to benefit ratios. For example, the deontological position would be determined by deciding what is the morally correct thing to do. Kant's writings are synonymous with deontology and he asserted that the end can never justify the means (Kemp Smith, 1973). Such a position can be seen to be indicating the importance of non-maleficence. In terms of benefit to risk issues for ExCs, even if the outcome of the research was illustrated to have wide reaching benefits, if these can only be achieved by unethical research, then the research study is not justifiable or ethically sound.

In contrast, the utilitarian standpoint would be judged according to the outcome of the study (Thompson *et al*, 1988). Utilitarianists would consider, what is the greatest good for the greatest number of people. Such ethical positions are concerned with the outcome or consequence of the study and are grouped under the term con-sequentialism (Thompson *et al*, 1988). Such a position can be seen to indicate the importance of beneficence. In terms of benefit to risk ratio, a person with a consequentialist ethical standpoint may regard a study as ethically sound, even though some harm may befall some of the participants, if the outcomes/findings of the study are seen to benefit a greater number of people (Beauchamp and Childress, 1994).

Ethics committees have to balance the risk to benefit ratio in qualitative studies that propose to access ExCs and, in doing so, most often adopt the stance that the risks are inherent in the interview process and the benefits exist, largely, for the wider population and much less for the interviewees. Yet, it should be noted that such a position is not supported by an abundance of evidence and perhaps can be regarded as somewhat inappropriate.

Outcomes from participating in qualitative interviews: equivocal findings

The evidence that talking of one's experiences of counselling will produce uncomfortable emotions is equivocal. Munhall (1991) high-lights that for a participant, the experience of a qualitative interview can be emotionally charged and distressing for some, while for others it can be a validating and therapeutic experience. Furthermore, May (1991) described some of the ethical issues in qualitative interviewing and suggested that since interviews may stimulate self-reflection, appraisal or catharsis, and considerable self-disclosure, the investigator needs to take these possibilities into account and consider what provisions need to be made for the informant's well being. Additionally, there is a large body of theory and empirical evidence that alludes to the potential therapeutic value of telling one's story and being listened to (for example, see Rogers, 1952; Peplau, 1952; Egan, 1975). Indeed, in the largest study of users' appreciation of psychiatric services in the UK, Rogers et al (1993) found that a preferred model of practice involved personal contact and understanding, being listened and responded to empathetically.

Usher and Holmes (1997) declared that during qualitative research interviews, the relationship between the researcher/participant can range from civil co-operation to therapeutic alliance. They further argue that since the participants are on 'home turf' they are often more knowledgeable than the researcher and thus the power base changes. Therefore, while accessing experiences of counselling may evoke painful feelings, it is also possible that telling their story of the counselling experience may be therapeutic for the ExCs and could be regarded as a beneficent act.

Raudonis (1992) argued that there is danger in qualitative researchers erring on the side of caution and being over protective of potentially vulnerable participants. Due to the emergent nature of the design of qualitative studies, all potential risks to the participants may not be known. Similarly, all potential benefits to the participants may not be known. In Raudonis' (1992) study, to determine hospice patients' perspectives of nurse empathy, only one person stated that they did not have the energy to participate and declined the invitation. Raudonis reported that all the other fourteen participants reported benefiting from their involvement. One participant stated:

... and I'm glad to do it [participate in the study] because I don't get a chance to help people much anymore. They're helping me, you know. So, its nice to be able to do that.

(Raudonis, 1992, p. 242)

It should be noted that fourteen respondents in one study cannot be taken to be representative of all potentially vulnerable participants and it would be unwise to base an argument on this one study. However, during her key note presentation at the fifth qualitative health research conference in Newcastle, Australia, and in personal correspondence with Professor Janice Morse following this presentation, she stated that in her extensive qualitative research experience, she has never had a participant who has reported that the experience of being interviewed was harmful. She further adds:

*Review committees sometimes express concern that the interview process may be stressful to some participants. This is not generally the case, even though the participants may become upset during the interview. They generally express appreciation that someone has **at last listened** [original emphasis] to their stories.*

(Morse and Field, 1995, p. 93)

Morse and Field (1995) note that the interview can sometimes be the first opportunity the clients have had to tell it all and that this in itself gives interviewees an opportunity to put it all together. An argument supported by Norris (1991) who discovered similar responses when she interviewed mothers who had given consent for their daughter's abortion. Norris noted that even though the mothers became quite upset during the interview, by the time they had finished they were laughing and joking. Norris pointed out that the interview itself was a cathartic experience, enabling the mothers to talk about these issues and relieve their distress in a way that they could not do even with their husbands. Morse and Field (1995) conclude that the qualitative interview may be a very therapeutic experience. Consequently, perhaps Raudonis' (1992, p. 242) arguments regarding ethical concerns in qualitative research have substance when she states:

> *In protecting the patients' human rights regarding participation in research, a patient may be prevented from or restricted in exercising his or her right to self-determination.*

And that consequently:

> *Healthcare providers must tread a fine line between appropriately protecting vulnerable populations and paternalistic decision making supposedly made in the patient's best interest.*

Evaluative client feedback data on the experience of being interviewed

It is reasonable to suggest that the relevant theoretical and empirical literature is not replete with unequivocal findings that demonstrate the therapeutic benefit of participating in a qualitative interview. Neither is it the purpose of this chapter to provide such evidence. However, as illustrated in the previous section, such evidence is starting to emerge (Norris, 1991; Raudonis, 1992; Morse and Field, 1995). In keeping with Professor Morse's experience, having conducted qualitative research studies for over eight years, all of which included the use of interviews as a means of data collection, the author has never encountered an interviewee who was re-traumatised by the experience. This led the author to consider attempting to obtain some feedback from ex-clients who had participated in the interviews. The next section of this chapter provides some evaluative feedback from the ex-clients who consented to participate in a study that looked at the inspiration of hope in bereavement counselling. All of the ex-clients consented not only to be interviewed for that study, but additionally, to provide feedback on the experience of being interviewed. All the names mentioned in the interviews have been changed.

First interview

Interviewer (I):   Perhaps now if you could tell me something about the process of being interviewed.

Respondent (R):   Well, it was pretty much as I expected it would be. Although I was a little surprised by it.

I: Could you say a little bit more about that.

R: Yes. After we had spoken on the phone (prior to the interview), I thought about what the interview would be like. For some reason I thought that it would be a lot more questions and answers. You know, short questions and quick answers. So I guess I was surprised by how little you said. I imagined you might have a clipboard and tick boxes. I mean, I knew that we would be talking about the loss of Bret, but the interview felt more reflective than I thought it would.

I: How comfortable was that reflection?

R: Well that's what I mean. As I thought about and talked about Bret's death, several things became apparent to me. I am aware that I am trying to make sense of the loss, maybe understand it a bit more, and what helps me with that, in some small way, is knowing that my experience can maybe help someone else. You know, Bret would want that. He was a very generous person, always giving. He loved it when he could share his toys with his sister, so I know he would want to help other people, even in this. And knowing that, knowing that other people may not have to go through what I have had to go through, that somehow makes it easier. I'm not saying its easy or that this is something I force. It is more a case that this became evident to me as I talked about my loss.

I: So let me just check out that I understand, the interview has helped you in ways you did not expect. That somehow in talking about your experiences, you have found something that you didn't realise.

R: Almost. I think I have known for a while, but I haven't been conscious of it for a while. So yes, talking about it like this has reminded me of it. Also, as someone who has benefited from therapy, I understand the need for therapy. What I mean is, I understand that it is necessary to develop therapy. Therapy can't stand still and the therapists need to learn. So this sort of thing (the research) needs to occur.

I: Thank you, I think that covers it.

Second interview

I: So, if we could move onto the feedback, how did the interview feel?

R: It was ok. It goes very quickly, doesn't it?

I: Yes, indeed. Would you like to say some more?

R: Sure, when you actually get into it, you just focus on what you are thinking and feeling, and about what questions are asked. I felt more guarded or unsafe at the start, but that diminished as time went on.

I: I'm glad about that. What about the subject matter, was it painful to talk about?

R: Well yes, it wasn't easy, but then it never is talking about my mother. But that shouldn't stop me. You know, I want to talk about her, keep the memory alive, keep her as part of my life. I think it would be very wrong if I stopped thinking or talking about her and it is funny in a way because not everyone is comfortable with this.

I: What do you mean?

R: It's just that it seems that not everyone is comfortable talking about, or hearing others talking about, death or bereavement. So, I don't get the chance to talk about my mother very much. Even some of those people who are close to me, people who also knew her. It is a bit like they don't want to see me upset, or can't handle it if I'm upset. So they steer clear of mentioning her.

I: Is there a sense of you benefiting from the interview then?

R: That would depend on the individual. But in my case, yes, there was a benefit.

I: Did you feel able to say 'no', when you were asked if you would participate?

R: Certainly, I didn't feel pressured.

I: And during the interview did you feel you could stop at any time?

R: I suppose so, but it never occurred to me.

I: That's fine, thank you

Third interview

I: Thanks for that, if we could now focus on the interview itself. What did it feel like?

R: It was pretty much like I expected. As I told you at the start, I don't have a problem talking about my loss.

I: Could you say a bit more about that please?

R: Yes, sure. Ever since I completed my therapy, or should I say stopped going to therapy because I know there is an argument that says you never complete. Anyway, since I stopped going I haven't talked about the loss much. Not because it was too painful to do so, but because I didn't feel the need to.

I: I see.

R: I suppose it makes sense really. I wouldn't have stopped going to the therapy if I still needed to work on the issues. That would have been premature. To stop going before I had done what I needed to do. So, it was not difficult and I didn't expect it to be.

I: Ah ha.

R: In some ways, the experience of this interview confirms what I was saying.

I: What do you mean by that?

R: Well, we have talked about the loss, the therapy, the counsellor, you know, quite deep stuff. But none of it has upset me. So, this indicates progress to me, that I can still talk about these things without getting upset. It kind of confirms that I ended the therapy at the right time.

I: So, what would have happened if you had finished your therapy prematurely, and then agreed to participate in this interview?

R: That is difficult to answer because it is not my experience. However, for me personally, if it became apparent to me, as a result of the interview, that I still needed to go to therapy, then I would go back to therapy. But that wouldn't be a bad thing, would it?

I: I'm not sure what you mean.

R: I don't think having therapy is a bad thing and similarly, I don't think becoming aware that I need therapy then is also a bad thing. So, if I find out that I still have some issues then I don't see that as a problem of the interview.

I: Let me just check out that I understand. Hypothetically, prior to an interview you are unaware that you have unresolved issues. After the interview you realise that you do have issues and need to go back to therapy, has the interview done you some harm?

R: I would say no, because the interview didn't cause the harm, it just made you aware of the harm. You know, you have already suffered the loss, that wasn't the interview. Some people may prefer not to know, but for me, I have never believed that ignorance is bliss.

I: That's fine, thank you.

Fourth interview

I: So, just to finish off, I would like to ask you about the interview itself, how was it?

R   Fine.

I: Has it caused you harm in any way?

R: I don't think so.

I: What about talking about painful issues?

R: Well, if I didn't want to talk about such things then I could have said 'no' to the interview.

I: And were you able to do that?

R: Of course, but I have reasons for agreeing.

I: Such as?

I: Well one is wanting some good to come out of Sid's death.

I: I see.

R: Talking about his death is necessary. That's what the counselling was all about. So why should I be bothered about the idea of talking about the counselling? That's perhaps where some good can come from this.

I: What would you say then if someone had not allowed you to make the decision about participating?

R: What do you mean?

I: If someone or somebody had decided that as a member of a 'vulnerable group', it would be unfair to ask you to participate?

R: I would say that's not right. You know, I am a big girl. I make my own decisions and I can easily say 'No'.

I: Thank you.

Qualitative research interviews and matters of empowerment

Examination of these four sets of feedback indicates that there appeared to be an element of explicit benefit for each of the ExCs. These benefits include:

- a desire to see others benefiting from their experience
- the hope that as a result of learning from this experience, others may be spared some of the pain
- a clear element of being able to 'tell their story', and for that matter, the story of the deceased as it was their story too
- a sense of honouring the memory of the deceased
- a sense of confirming the sense of progress that the ExC had made
- a sense of closure
- a sense of giving something back, hoping that some 'good' could come from the loss.

Importantly, not one of the ExCs found talking about the experience traumatic.

It is important to note that often one aim of counselling is concerned with emancipation, freeing clients to take more control of their own lives and empower them. It can be regarded as somewhat paradoxical then for clients to undergo an emancipatory process, only then for the same people to be denied the right to self-determination in any subsequent qualitative research study. It can additionally be regarded as more inappropriate to deny ExCs the option of consenting/not consenting to a research process, which may in itself provide them with the opportunity for further therapeutic experience (and catharsis if they need it).

Safeguards and 'safety nets'

Having touched upon the emerging arguments within the literature, and provided some tentative evidence from ex-clients, it is important to note that it would be naïve to suggest that qualitative research interviews do not present ethical issues, and consequently it would be prudent of qualitative researchers to consider the possibility that their interview may cause harm. In order to maximise the potential for the qualitative interview to become a therapeutic or beneficent act, the researcher should seek ways to prevent/minimise harm and provide safeguards and safety nets. *Figure 13.1* provides a summary of the possible antecedents of harm to ex-clients who agree to be interviewed for a qualitative research study.

---

1.   Being identified as an ex-client, breach of confidentiality boundaries and the possible stigmatisation that could accompany this (Etherington, 1996).
2.   The production of uncomfortable feelings that could be evoked as a result of speaking of their experience of counselling (McLeod, 1996; Usher and Holmes, 1997).
3.   The possible exploitation of, arguably, vulnerable people (Grafanaki, 1996; Etherington, 1996).

Figure 13.1: Possible antecedents of harm to participating ex-clients

In response to the first of these potential antecedents to harm, the qualitative researcher might want to consider the use of an intermediary. Achieving access to ex-clients without any breach of confidentiality occurring is a difficult process. One such method involves contacting the ex-clients through an intermediary, preferably an individual who is already known to the ex-client. Perhaps the counsellors who provided the therapy to the clients can operate in this role, and introductory letters, information sheets and any other appropriate literature could be passed on via the counsellor to the ex-clients. Any individual who does not wish to be identified as an ex-client need not respond to the initial contact letter. For those individuals who do respond to the initial contact letter, a response appears to indicate that they had no problem with being identified to the researcher as an ex-client. The researcher would then need to assure the ex-client that the identity of each individual who is willing to participate would be known only to the researcher and his supervisor, assuring these individuals of their complete confidentiality. Consequently, no harm to ex-clients would result from identifying themselves to the researcher as an ex-client.

In response to the second of these potential antecedents to harm, two *modus operandi* are suggested. Firstly, the possibility of individuals who agreed to participate in the study accessing painful emotions should be made clear in the information sheet. If any individuals feel this potential was too much of a threat, then they simply need not reply or consent to be interviewed. Secondly, for any individuals who agreed to participate in the study and find that the experience of being interviewed accesses painful emotions, a 'safety net' of counselling services that they could use should be made available. All participants should be aware of this information prior to being interviewed.

In response to the third of these potential antecedents to harm, Grafanaki (1996) and Etherington (1996) both illustrated the potentially vulnerable position counselling clients are in. The argument about possible harm occuring from discussing painful material has been acknowledged, however, questions should be asked about whether or not ex-clients have the same degree of vulnerability as current clients. The issues of vulnerability and exploitation within a research study for current counselling clients centre around the sense of being coerced into agreeing to participate (McLeod, 1996; Grafanaki, 1996; Etherington, 1996). Individuals may believe that failure to comply will somehow affect the counselling they receive or alter the dynamics of the relationship between themselves and the counsellor. If these arguments are considered for ex-clients it becomes clear that concerns of exploitation are not well-founded. Since the ex-client would not be receiving any therapy, this counselling could not be affected by not agreeing to participate. Similarly, since there is no current relationship between ex-client and counsellor, the dynamics cannot be affected.

In summary

Current practice of ethics committees in deciding whether or not to grant approval to qualitative research studies appears to contain an element of paternalism. This may or may not be a laudable ethical position to adopt, but there is growing argument which suggests that such deliberations need to take more account of the evidence that indicates the possible benefits of the process of the study, not the outcomes. While there is evidence to indicate that these benefits appear to be wide and varied, they are a 'secondary gain' or a 'bonus', not the primary purpose of research interviews.

The sometimes over-paternalistic decisions of ethics committees may be particularly inappropriate for ExCs, where the emphasis is on empowering the client, emancipation and increased personal autonomy, since there is an element of counselling practice that is concerned with helping people take more control of their own lives. If healthcare practitioners are genuinely concerned with client empowerment and participation, then it can be regarded as somewhat pompous and arrogant of us, as members of ethics committees, to decide what is in the person's best interest without giving the person the opportunity to say for themselves.

Of course, these are somewhat preliminary thoughts and undeveloped arguments that have been used purposefully to illustrate the point. In no way is the author suggesting that issues of consent and participation and access to clients for qualitative interviews are simple, straightforward and do not deserve much consideration. For example, additional issues such as how the approach is made, who makes the approach, and avoiding any sense of coercion must be considered. If ethics committees are undertaking comprehensive consideration and genuinely representing the interests of the public and people, then they need to give due consideration of this other variable: the empowering, beneficial and therapeutic effects of engaging in qualitative research interview.

Key points

* Local research ethics committees (LRECs) have a duty of care to promote research which enables both participant and researcher. The values on which decisions are made should be considered in their own right, to determine to what extent paternalism has influenced them.

* Concern is expressed that intermediary bodies such as ethic committees are able to decide on consent issues for third parties, and participation in the research process does not automatically cause the participant harm.

* Participant feedback is important to evaluate the process. The ex-clients who were interviewed for this chapter seemed to have gained some explicit benefits from the process, yet this type of positive feedback is rarely taken into account by LRECs who continue to make over-paternalistic decisions in blind good faith.

* Sometimes over-paternalistic decisions made by LRECs may be inappropriate, undermine emancipation and the clients who participate. There are empowering, beneficial and therapeutic effects of engaging in a qualitative research interview.

References

Beauchamp TL, Childress JF (1994) *Principles of Biomedical Ethics.* 4th edn. Oxford University Press, Oxford

Cartwright A (1998) *Health surveys in practice and potential: A critical review of their scope and methods.* King's Fund, London

Department of Health (1991) *Local Research Ethics Committees.* DoH, London

Department of Health (1994) *Local Research Ethics Committees: A Framework for ethical review.* DoH, London

Egan G (1975) *The Skilled Helper.* Aldine, Chicago

Etherington K (1996) The counsellor as researcher: Boundary issues and critical dilemmas. *Br J Guidance Counselling* **24**(3): 339–46

Garritson SH, Davis AJ (1983) Least restrictive alternative. *J Psychosoc Nurs* **21**(12): 17–23

Grafanaki S (1996) How research can change the researcher: The need for sensitivity, flexibility and ethical boundaries in conducting qualitative research in counselling/psychotherapy. *Br J Guidance Counselling* **24**(3): 329–38

Kemp Smith N, translator (1973) *Immanuel Kant's Critique of Pure Reason.* Macmillan, London

Lasagna L (1970) Special subjects in human experimentation. In: Freund PA *Experimentation with Human Subjects.* Allen & Unwin, Sydney: 262–75

Lipson JG (1994) Ethical issues in ethnography. In: Morse JM, ed. *Critical Issues in Qualitative Research Methods.* Sage, London: 333–55

McLeod J (1996) Qualitative approaches to research in counselling and psychotherapy: Issues and challenges. *Br J Guidance Counselling* **24**(3): 309–16

May KA (1991) Interviewing techniques in qualitative research: concerns and challenges. In: Morse JM, ed. *Qualitative Nursing Research: a contemporary dialogue.* Sage, Newbury Park: 187–201

Morse JM, Field PA (1995) *Qualitative Research Methods for Healthcare Professionals.* 2nd edn. Sage, London

Munhall PL (1991) Institutional review of qualitative research proposals: a task of no small consequence. In: Morse JM, ed. *Qualitative Nursing Research: a contemporary dialogue.* Sage, Newbury Park: 258–71

Norris J (1991) Mother's involvement in their adolescent daughters' abortions. In: Morse JM, Johnson JL, eds. *The Illness experience: Dimensions of suffering.* Sage, London: 201–36

Peplau HE (1952) *Interpersonal Relations in Nursing.* Macmillan, London

Raudonis BM (1992) Ethical considerations in qualitative research with hospice patients. *Qualitative Health Res* **2**(2): 238–49

Rogers C (1952) *Client Centred Therapy: Its current practice, implications and theory.* Constable, London

Rogers A, Pilgrim D, Lacey R (1993) *Experiencing Psychiatry: Users views of services.* Macmillan/ MIND, London

Royal College of Physicians (1990) *Guidelines on the practice of ethics committees in medical research involving human subjects.* The Royal College of Physicians, London

Royal College of Physicians (1996) *Guidelines on the practice of ethics committees in medical research involving human subjects.* The Royal College of Physicians, London

Thompson IE, Melia KM, Boyd KM (1988) *Nursing Ethics.* 2nd edn. Churchill Livingstone, Edinburgh

Usher K, Holmes C (1997) Ethical aspects of phenomenological research with mentally ill people. *Nurs Ethics* **4**(1): 49–56

Watson AB (1982) Informed consent of special subjects. *Nurs Res* **31**: 43–7

World Medical Association (1964) *Declaration of Helsinki.* World Medical Association, South Africa

14

Empowerment and participation: the arts in health care

Larry Butler

> *Whatever you can do or dream you can do, begin it!*
> *Boldness has genius, magic and power in it. Begin it now!*

(Goethe)

Sing it. Paint it. Write it. Play it. Tell it. Mould it. Act it. Mime it. Dance it. Whatever **it** is: pain, feeling, dreams, hopes, fears; using your imagination, you can transform it into something else exuding truth, beauty, and maybe, even health and well-being. The arts can and do make a difference in many people's lives. However, the Stockport Arts and Health leaflet states:

> *The arts are central to human life... and yet sadly, in our society actually doing art is too often neglected and left to the professionals.*

All the arts have proved to be excellent vehicles for people who experience mental distress to regain a sense of self-worth and a new purpose in life (Brown, 1977).

Over the past forty years, there has been a growing body of literature about the excellent work being done in the fields of art, drama and music therapy. This chapter will focus on a few of the many individual artists, and arts organisations throughout the UK who promote the arts in health care, empowering clients and patients.

How do we know the arts can help?

We don't. As yet, there is very little scientific evidence to justify the use of arts in health care. Participation in creative activities may act as a key to helping people communicate more effectively, and engage in wider social activities. Research carried out in Manchester (Bridges *et al*, 1991) has shown that people discharged from psychiatric hospitals have fewer re-admissions when attending the START

Studios. Evidence suggests that art, and particularly the participation in art, may result in savings to the health and social services (Bridges and Brown, 1989).

According to the recent review *Arts for Health* carried out by the Health Education Authority, 'the number of community-focused projects and initiatives which use the arts to impact health and well-being has risen rapidly during the last decade' (SHM Productions Ltd). In another report commissioned by the Scottish Arts Council to explore the role of the arts in healthy living centres, it is stated that:

> *There is scope to promote the notion of the arts as a means of self-expression and as a catalyst for strengthening and energising communities and enhancing the psychological, physical and emotional health and well-being of the individuals who make up those communities.*

> (Troup, 1999)

The Comedia Report, *The Art of Regeneratio*, highlights the contribution of the arts to the development of human potential:

> *Those working to renew our cities accept that wealth creation, social cohesion, and quality of life ultimately depend on confident, imaginative citizens who feel empowered and are able to fulfil their potential. And they have turned increasingly to the arts as a mechanism to trigger individual and community development*

> (Landrey, 1996, p. 2)

In March 1998, *Arts on Prescription* (Dalton and Mackenzie-Reid, 1998) was launched as a national campaign, 'to enhance public health and well-being into the twenty-first century'. This was initiated by a high level group of doctors, academics, artists, healthcare practitioners, and community development leaders, spearheaded by the then Chief Medical Officer for England and Wales, Sir Kenneth Calman, who has gone on to establish the Centre for the Arts and Humanities in Health and Medicine (CAHHM) at Durham University. Another member of this group, Dr Robin Philipp, University of Bristol, states:

> *We spend £81 million a year in Britain on anti-depressants, and the cost per patient can be as high as £300 a year. If we can wean just a few of these patients off*

such drugs through the use of arts in health care, then it will be worth it.

CAHHM considers that the benefits likely to arise from the use of the arts in complementing scientific and technological modes of diagnosis and treatment include:

- more compassionate, intuitive doctors and other health practitioners
- an essential aid in combating social exclusion
- reduced dependence on anti-depressant prescription drugs
- patient empowerment through creative expression
- growing confidence and self-reliance of individuals and communities.

> The Centre for the Arts and Humanities in Health and Medicine (CAHHM) was established in January 2000 with the aim of improving the quality of community health and of the lives of individual patients and health professionals. CAHHM seeks to improve the knowledge of health professionals about the role of arts in health by developing a high quality evidence base.

When a feasibility study for *Arts on Prescription* in Glasgow was discussed with the famous clown doctor Patch Adams, he said: 'It's a pity you have to prove something that is so obvious'. However, as indicated in the *Arts for Health* review:

> *To date there is no single sound and established set of principles and protocols for evaluating outcomes, assessing the processes by which outcomes are achieved and disseminating recommendations for good practice to workers in the field.*

> (SHM Productions Ltd, 1999)

There is a need for rigorous evaluation and action research, which brings together artists and healthcare practitioners and participants.

What's on offer and who is doing what?

There are many agencies promoting the arts in health care (see

'Useful organisations', *p. 257*). Some artists specialise in the people they work with, some specialise in the art forms they offer. People are being empowered to participate in the arts to help themselves. For example, patients in the Glasgow's Western Infirmary are encouraged to listen to music in preparation for an operation and help relieve pain. After a school bus crashed in the Midlands, killing and injuring many children, the families, teachers and friends have gathered regularly to share stories, write poems and make pictures which has helped them come to terms with their loss and re-build their community. This was facilitated by a local poet and a storyteller. The following descriptions and quotes aim to give you a flavour of the range of creative activities offered in health care around the UK.

'Poet for health' residency at Dean lane family practice, Bristol (Flint, 2000)

Rose Flint worked one day a week for six months in this busy practice of 9,200 patients served by six resident doctors. The project was initiated by one of the resident general practitioners and funded by the Poetry Places Scheme. Ms Flint found it difficult to describe her role. What she and one of the doctors agreed was the following brief: 'using poetry as a way of helping people to engage with their emotions'. This placed the emphasis on the process of writing, not the product.

So, what did she do? She designed a poster for the waiting room which stated:

> Tell it how it is — Your life... Your health... Your voice
> Every Tuesday, Poet for Health, Rose Flint, will be in the surgery offering one hour poetry sessions to anyone who would like to explore the way they feel through the creative medium of words
> For more information please ask one of the receptionists, nurses or doctors.

Patients could be referred by their doctor or practice nurse or self-refer by simply asking the reception staff to book an appointment. Dr Rice and Ms Flint selected dozen of poems for display in the waiting rooms, and piles of photocopies of other poems with an invitation to 'please take one'. The piles magically disappeared and were regularly replenished, themes of the poems changing with the seasons. Ms Flint writes in her report: 'the poems themselves, their presence and mass felt like an ally for me'. All her clients expressed the need to 'talk' as a priority:

Working with words, I found that the 'material' would be, in effect, the words spoken between us, everything that the client brought to the session and my response.

(Flint, 2000)

Here are some comments by a woman who saw Ms Flint individually and in a group. She is over-weight and has osteoarthritis and bouts of depression:

Writing helps me deal with my problems. I wrote about abusive boys. Writing stops me from going to the fridge or buying a bar of chocolate. I've lost over a stone. With this writing-lark, I can let flow from my head down my arm onto the paper... I can see the leaves and the fruit on the trees because I wrote about my anger.

Another woman said: 'coming to the writer's group has helped me not see my GP. And I've stopped taking my anti-depressants.'

Early on in the residency, Rose dropped the idea that there would be a huge production of poetry. This raised many questions for her, about what poetry actually is: 'Sylvia Plath once said that poetry was her "deepest health". Yeats called poetry, "the voice of the soul"... poetry has within it the desire for life.'

All the participants gave very good feedback. One person wrote:

I think this programme is very effective and for me, a life-saver. My writing also helped me to take my mind off my pain.

Everyone, staff and participants, felt that the time was too short and this has been a problem with many arts in healthcare projects. But there is one project, which seems to have lasted and grown organically over many years, the Bromley-by-Bow Healthy Living Centre.

Bromley-by-Bow Healthy Living Centre

With windows and skylights, high ceilings and surrounded by sculpture and paintings, sitting in the waiting area, you feel better before you even see the doctor. Here are the partnerships between the National Health Service, complementary therapies, local authorities, church, the business community and the arts. 'There is more to improving health than prescriptions' seems to be their motto (BMA Review, 1998, pp. 38–39). The facilities and services include: an education programme, exercise on prescription, a community café, a park, a herb and vegetable garden, adventure play area, sculpture studio, pottery, textile and painting studios, a nursery, a crèche, a music room, creative writing, literacy, yoga, aromatherapy and more.

A woman, who was mopping the floor of the large multi-purpose hall after she had worked as a volunteer during a visual art workshop with fifty people (twenty-five volunteers, twenty-five people with a disability) was also the local minister and a director of the centre. This seems to be how Bromley-by-Bow works, everyone gets involved and everyone has a say. One of the GPs, Dr Sam Everington, says most of the projects were started by patients, who improved their health and job prospects in the process. A BMA review describes the centre as:

A jewel in an East London sea of congested roads and tower blocks, Bromley-by-Bow is seen as the prototype for the government's healthy living centres.

(British Medical Association Review, 1998, pp. 38–39)

Stockport Arts and Health

This is an NHS funded scheme to enhance the social and physical environment for health care in Stockport by means of the arts. They promote patient, staff and community involvement in the arts. They facilitate creative activity as a means of communication, empowerment, and healthy living for the people of Stockport.

This work is done by commissioning artists to work with groups in hospitals and in the community, in making artworks for health venues. One of their projects is called RAP! (Reminiscence Arts Project) and includes storytelling, creative writing, silk painting, music and partying. Stockport Arts on Prescription (AoP) is another project which:

> *... offers the arts as a means of restoring mental well-being whilst feelings of distress are relatively manageable — with the intention of preventing the need for admission to mainstream mental health services.*

Activities include; craft workshops, drama, creative writing, visual art, and Qigong (a Chinese form of relaxation). Here are some comments from AoP participants:

> *I can be myself more... It's a great way to relax and forget about your problems... I was nervous at first and didn't think I could write — by the end of the session I'd written a poem... I feel it's brilliant, I never want the sessions to end... It was great to see that I had achieved something at the end of two hours... Here I can concentrate on being creative. At home I start thinking, worrying, can't concentrate and the worrying stops me doing things...*

> (Stockport Arts Newsletter, 1996)

Patients are referred by their GP, who simply fills out a prescription pad which is sent to the project. A visit is then arranged by the project manager (who is a community mental health nurse). Sometimes there have been inappropriate referrals for individuals who are too depressed, or have recently left hospital. After ten weeks there is a review. As well as enjoying the creative activity and social company, the participants report that it increases the amount of other activities they do elsewhere (Stockport Arts on Prescription, 1999).

Survivors' Poetry

This is a national literature and performance organisation dedicated to promoting poetry by survivors of mental distress through workshops, performances, reading, and publications to audiences all over the UK. In a recent newsletter, one member writes:

> *Poetry has not only purged my system and helped channel debilitating depression, it has given me a new lease of life.*

> (Hurst, 2000, p. 6–7)

Since Survivors' Poetry was founded in 1991 by four poets with first-hand experience of the mental health system, they have supported the formation of a nationwide network of survivors' writing groups and work in partnership with local and national arts, mental health, community and disability organisations. These groups have managed to combine artistic expression with advocacy and empowerment. Although some of their activities on stage, in workshops and publications may well be therapeutic, they claim that their purpose, is quality communication and 'celebrating who we are in all our diversities, and to encourage all survivors to come out, and speak out with pride, dignity and beauty'.

Here is a poem by Susan Watters (1996), a member of a group in Glasgow. Her poem was published and performed many times, as part of a revue touring hospitals.

A patient's life in the day of a psychiatric nurse

Get off that bed!

I don't care if you're tired. Just do
what you're told and get off the bed.

You're not going to leave that bed
in that mess. Straighten it up!

No, you can't go for a walk,
you haven't got a ground pass.

Just go and sit in the day hall
and watch some television.

Don't take that cup into the ward,
you only drink in the day hall.

No, you can't have something for a headache,
the doctor says you haven't got one.

I'm not turning the radio down,
the other patients like it loud.

That doesn't matter, they'll be back soon
and don't you answer me back, madam!

And don't go getting any ideas
about lying on your bed again.

I don't care whether you like it or not,
just eat it!

Switch off that television
and get into bed!

Susan wrote a song which was performed in call and response to the style of an American Sergeant major:

> We are crazy, we are mad
> Sometimes good, sometimes bad
> Ain't no doctor going to detain me
> Cause I got six personalities
> Whichever one he locks up
> The other five will be running a muck
> So doctor why don't you leave us
> poor crazy people alone
> For we are crazy, we are maaaad!

After singing this song at a conference in Dunblane about the hospital closure programme in the presence of senior healthcare professionals, Survivors' Poetry was encouraged to start a new group in Lothian.

Here is another poem expressing a different sentiment by Peter Campbell (1996), one of the founders of Survivors' Poetry:

That pleasure

> There is a pleasure madmen know
> After the bath.
> As they stand in the arms of their beltless clothes
> And the scrutineers have left the room
> with a practised laugh.
> There is that pleasure then.
>
> There is a pleasure madmen know
> After dusk.
> As they search for gods in the pewter skies
> And the scrutineer lays down Jane Eyre
> Beside his desk.
> There is that pleasure then.
>
> There is a pleasure madmen know
> of their kind.
> As they embrace by the pot room door
> and the scrutiny of the caring crowd
> Has gone blind.
> There is that pleasure then.
>
> There is a pleasure madmen know
> Without the wine —-
> That blood and reason hang themselves
> On the same line
> And the scrutineers dispense love
> For the last time.
> There is that pleasure then.

There is a pleasure sure
In being mad, which none but madmen know!

(John Dryden)

Art in hospital

Dotted around the UK, there are a growing number of projects dedicated to bringing visual arts into health care. The Glasgow Art in Hospital is based at Blawarthill Hospital, and employs eleven part-time staff working in six hospitals. They involve patients in a diverse range of art activities, supported and supplemented with music, books, slides and photographs, as well as a programme of outside visits to Glasgow's museums and galleries. Their approach is designed to meet the specific needs of each individual, encouraging them to explore and develop their own creativity. They are committed to developing a framework for monitoring and evaluation, in order to measure the impact of the work. Their exhibition programme brings the artwork created by project participants to a wider audience, and also aims to 'humanise' and transform hospital environments (Gulliver, 1999).

This next poem was written and sung loudly to a friend in hospital recovering from a colostomy. The patient had been feeling depressed for days and embarrassed by the rumblings from the hole in his side. While listening to this song, he began to smile and laugh for the first time since his operation. The whole ward was in an uproar — the visitor came in singing, dressed like a tramp and pretending to be drunk!

Sick Song for Robert Kimble

(very slow sleepy blues, each verse repeated twice or more while yawning)

> Got a fever
> and a cold
> oh I must
> be gettin old
>
> I'm sick to death of diing
> I'm sick to death of diing
>
> Can't bend or bounce
> Can't bend or bounce

so I must rest
or I might rust
in a puddle
growing watercress
on my belly

I'm sick to death of diing
I'm sick to death of diing

Or ah might curdle in a corner
Or ah might curdle in a corner
snuggle under cover
huggle heavy sights
quiet coos be snoozing

I'm sick to death of diing
I'm sick to death of diing

So I'll jist lie still
So I'll jist lie still
and listen to my orifices
emit loud smelly sounds

I'm sick to death of diing
I'm sick to death of diing

All too slow
All too slow
I gotta get well
or I'll get worse

I'm sick to death of diing
I'm sick to death of diing
I'm sick to death of diing

During the hospital visit was written by a father-to-be, when he was waiting outside while his pregnant wife was being examined. He was angry because the doctor would not allow him to attend the consultation.

During the hospital visit

During the hospital visit
our baby squirms in your belly
What can I do, I want to fly
away? Will *it* survive, be ok
die young?

I could climb mountains
while I wait, our child squirms
in your belly but maybe *it's* a lie

not the sky heavy with traffic smell —
will it ever come (come n go my
    dream of clean air n

easy to write poems) our baby
squirms in your belly, my father
retired from General Electric after
producing billions of pellets of uranium —
    they gave him a clock.

Already separate the pain's not
within me, our baby squirms in
your belly while my feet outside
stamp on concrete. I want to scream
    but the pain's not within me —
n your breasts grow big!

A recent study of the use of therapeutic writing in primary care, concluded that it is feasible for GPs and acceptable to patients (Hannay and Bolton, 1999). The doctors felt that therapeutic writing was beneficial to the patients, and could be incorporated into normal consultations with the use of explanatory leaflets. Here are the patient guidelines for therapeutic writing:

Whatever you write is right
Whatever you write is right
You can't write the wrong thing!
It doesn't even have to be in proper English.

This writing is only for you to read, at first.
You might want to reread it later, share it
with a relative, friend, some with your GP;
or even tear it up!

It may seem odd at first, writing like this.
rite when and where you feel like it: day
or night, in bed, in a café (difficult on a bike)

Write only two lines, or lots in a notebook
on scraps of paper, perhaps in a folder.

1. Scribble whatever comes into your head for 6 minutes
— don't stop to think!
— it might be a list. Or odd words or phrases
— spelling and proper sentences don't matter!

Therapeutic writing can be introduced with a simple explanatory leaflet (below) of patients' guidelines; it does not interfere with doctor-patient relationships and need not be time-consuming for doctors.

Either: Carry on or... Write about: a dream, a memory, a time of loss...

Or: Make a list of all the important people in your life. It doesn't matter if they are alive or dead now.

Choose one to describe. What did they say?
Write a letter as if you were talking to them.

This way of working/playing with writing could be adapted for other creative activities such as singing, dancing, drawing, painting, and playing with clay. Exercise on Prescription has become increasingly popular among patients and healthcare professionals throughout the UK. So why not the arts too? Doctors act as gatekeepers primarily for pharmaceutical and surgical interventions. With little additional cost, their role could be extended to empower many of their patients to be more expressive and creative in their everyday lives.

Conclusion

Is it therapy or is it art? And does it matter?

Although some of these projects target people who have suffered mental ill health, the arts are applicable and widely used across various areas of health care. For many years, there has been an ongoing debate about the arts as therapy versus the practice of the arts to promote better health. Can the arts be used like a medicine? Is there a danger that we might medicalise the arts? The Arts for Health review states that:

> *Participants in the best projects placed great emphasis on the importance of the quality of outcomes (eg. artworks) as well as the benefits of the process of involvement.*

> (SHM Productions Ltd, 1999)

The magic doesn't seem to work as well without the end product of an art work displayed, published, or performed.

In a letter to Dr Malcolm Rigler at the Withymoor Village Surgery, where for many years there has been a lively arts programme, Sir Kenneth Calman (1997) wrote:

> ... *it is fascinating to see health issues tackled in such a positive, friendly and enthusiastic way. In taking forward 'The Health of the Nation' strategy, one of the key features has been the development of partnerships and alliances at local level to meet health needs of the population... the Withymoor experience shows what can happen when you go beyond the traditional medical approach, to involve the arts in imaginative and exciting ways. Good fun is sometimes good medicine and the objective of the whole process is to improve quality of life for patients and the community .*

The Healthy Living Centre initiative gives renewed scope for the development of the application of the arts in health care. The number of community-focused projects which use the arts to impact health and well-being has risen rapidly during the last decade. There is an established body of good practice and research — local, national and international — which can provide initial evidence of the efficacy of the arts in promoting and maintaining good health and in effecting treatment. There is clearly a growing interest in a research and advocacy programme to develop arts in health care. This would have benefits for patients, arts and healthcare professionals, for the development of innovative approaches to health care, and for the health gain of the British people (Troup, 1999).

Key points

⌘ Despite 'very little scientific evidence to justify the use of arts in health care', research on service users' experiences suggests that therapeutic use of the arts make 'a difference to people's lives.' Benefits are emphasised in several reports, and in the national 'Arts on Prescription' campaign, launched in 1998.

⌘ Many organisations and services promote the arts in health care. These include a 'poet for health' residency at a family practice, a Healthy Living Centre, Stockport Arts and Health, Survivors' Poetry, and an Art in Hospital Project.

⌘ Benefits reported by participants include the expression of bereavement and difficult feelings, relieving pain and depression, enabling a sense of achievement, and developing and expressing creativity. A Healthy Living Centre improved patients' 'health and job prospects'. Survivors' Poetry aims to celebrate diversity, and enables coming out and speaking out, 'with pride, dignity and beauty'.

⌘ Poems included in the chapter illustrate a mental health nurse's authoritarian attitudes, and experiences of mental illness and a colostomy. An expectant father writes about his anger at a doctor's refusal to allow him to attend a consultation about his wife and their baby.

⌘ A recent study found that general practitioners considered therapeutic writing to be of benefit to patients. Patient guidelines for this writing have been devised.

⌘ 'Medicalisation of the arts' is a possible danger. One review found that the quality of art produced was as important to participants as the benefits of being involved.

⌘ The number of community-based Arts in Health projects has increased considerably in the last ten years. Examples of beneficial practice and positive research findings indicate that arts projects enable and promote good health and facilitate treatment. Further developments would benefit service users and other people.

References

Brown A (1997) *Stockport Arts and Health*. St Thomas' Hospital, Stockport

Bridges K, Brown L (1989) Psychiatric patients work alongside artist in prize-winning project. *Br Med J* **299**: 532

Bridges K, Brown L, Colgan S, Farragher B (1991) A tentative START in community care. *Psychiatric Bull* **15**: 596–8

British Medical Association (1998) *News Review*. May 16: 38 –39

Calman K (1997) Letter to Dr Malcolm Rigler, Withymoor Surgery: January

Campbell P (1996) *Sweet, Sour and Serious. Survivors' Poetry. Illustrated Anthology*. Survivors' Press, Glasgow: 16

Dalton R, Mackenzie-Reid D (1998) *Arts on Prescription: Campaign to improve the nation's health*. Windsor Conference sponsored by the Nuffield Trust

Flint R (2000) *Report: Poet for Health Residency*. Dean Lane Family Practice, Bristol

Gulliver J (1999) *Arts in Hospital leaflet*. Blawarthill Hospital, Glasgow

Hannay D, Bolton G (1999) Therapeutic writing in primary care. A feasibility study. *Primary Care Psychiatry* **5**: 157–60

Hurst J (2000) *When Poetry Rescued Me*. Survivors' Poetry Newsletter, March 7: 6–7

Landrey ET (1996) *The Art of Regeneration*. The Comedia Report: 2

SHM Productions Ltd (1999) *Arts for Health and Well-being*. Health Education Authority, London

Stockport Arts on Prescription (1999) *An Evaluation: The artists view*. May

Stockport Arts (1996) *Newsletter*. December

Troup M (1999) *Research and Advocacy for the Arts in Healthcare*. Scottish Arts Council, Edinburgh

Watters J (1996) *Sweet Sour and Serious. Survivors' Poetry Scotland. Illustrated Anthology*. Survivors' Press, Glasgow: 26

15

The power to complain?

Sue Evans and Richard Byrt

To what extent do NHS complaints procedures empower clients and patients and their informal carers and enable them to contribute to improvements in health care? This chapter attempts to answer this question, with reference to the literature and to developments in North Bristol NHS Trust.

'Complaints have been defined as expressions of dissatisfaction which require a response' (Stanton, 1997, p. 105). Allsop and Mulcahy state that, in relation to the NHS:

> *A 'complaint' may be taken as an expression of dissatisfaction which can be made orally or in writing. The dissatisfaction may be about the patient's own care or that received by someone else — a relative or a close friend.*

(Allsop and Mulcahy, 1995, p. 135)

The extent to which individual service users and carers feel able to complain, or to feel empowered or participate in their care, appears to depend, in part, on their relationships with service providers. Until the inception of the NHS, many people received free services as beneficiaries of charities or local parishes (Jones, 1993). Recipients were often expected to be grateful, rather than complain, an attitude criticised by Charles Dickens, and epitomised in the outraged reaction of Mr Bumble, the workhouse beadle, at Oliver Twist's 'asking for more' (Dickens, 1966).

From the late eighteenth century, a number of parliamentary and other reformers campaigned for improvements following the complaints of some asylum and workhouse inmates and their relatives. An example is Sarah Vickers, who in 1813, complained of the ill treatment of her husband in the asylum at York. Her complaint led to an investigation by a local reformer, Godfrey Higgins, which contributed to considerable reforms in local provision for people with mental illness (Jones, 1993).

The literature suggests that patients who pay for health services may be more likely to complain and to have relationships with doctors and other health professionals which are either equal, or with patients having control over decisions made (Friedson, 1975; Klein and Howlett, 1973). An extreme example of resolving a complaint concerns Astragaslide, a medieval French queen whose husband carried out her dying request to hurl her physician out of a window! (Friedson, 1975, quoting Reisman, 1935). However, high social status has often counted for nothing in people with mental health problems. The wishes and complaints of King George III were ignored by his doctors and attendants during his confinement with an apparent mental illness (MacAlpine and Hunter, 1969). John Perceval wrote of his treatment in an asylum in the eighteen thirties:

> *... I was never told, such and such things we are going to do; we think it advisable to administer such and such medicine. I was never asked have you any objection to this or that? My will, my wishes, my inclinations were not once consulted... I did not find the respect paid usually even to a child... the doctors... expunged from their consciences all deference to me; giving up so speedily and entirely all attempt at explanation...*

(Perceval, 1991; in Porter, 1991, p. 246,
first published in 1838/1840)

At the inception of the NHS in 1948, it was intended to establish systems for dealing with complaints, but these were not instituted because medical staff objected (Hogg, 1999, p. 32, citing Webster, 1996). The need for an inspectorate and for the systematic investigation of complaints became apparent following allegations, in the late nineteen-sixties and nineteen-seventies, of serious ill treatment and neglect of older people and individuals with learning disabilities and mental health problems. A succession of widely publicised scandals in hospitals resulted in the setting up of the Hospital (later, Health) Advisory Service (Hunt, 1995; Martin with Evans, 1984) and the Davies Committee, which 'recommended a national Code of Practice for dealing with suggestions and complaints about hospitals' (Hogg, 1999, p. 33). The NHS Reorganisation Act 1973 created the post of Health Service Commissioner or Ombudsman as (a supposedly independent) investigator of complaints in the NHS. Until 1996, the Health Service Commissioner could not investigate complaints about professionals' clinical judgement (Gunn, 2001; Limb, 1998).

The introduction of 'consumerism' in UK health services in the mid nineteen-eighties stressed the importance of the views of service users; and emphasised that they should have the same rights to complain as consumers of the services and products of free market organisations (Lupton *et al*, 1998). However, there is still some evidence that patients who complain are sometimes labelled 'difficult' (Duxbury, 2000).

Despite the recommendations of the Davies Committee, health services were not required to have complaints procedures until the Hospital Complaints Procedure Act 1985, was passed. Specific standards, related to this Act, were not specified by the Department of Health and Social Security at the time. 'A national complaints procedure for hospitals, community services and family practitioners was finally introduced in 1996' (Hogg, 1999, p. 33). This was based on the Wilson Review committee report on NHS complaints procedures, produced in May, 1994 (Department of Health, 1994); and 'Acting on Complaints', which included policy and proposals for a complaints procedure in England (Department of Health, 1995). *Guidance on Implementation of the NHS Complaints Procedure* produced by the NHS Executive in March 1996, included advice for managers and staff to enable them to help clients/patients and their carers to voice complaints. Feedback from complaints was intended to inform the development of improvements (National Health Service Executive, 1996).

Stages in the 1996 Complaints Procedure

At the time of writing this book, the 1996 Complaints Procedure is still operational within the NHS, but with plans for change, outlined on *p. 243*. There are four stages in the 1996 complaints procedure. In the first stage, 'local resolution', the complaint is investigated by a complaints manager, in line with the local complaints procedures, which vary between local health service organisations. Under the 1996 national complaints procedure, there are time limits for initial and final responses to complaints. The complaints manager may meet with the complainant and any staff or manager concerned. At this stage, external lay conciliators may be involved, acting 'as an intermediary between the complainant and the complained against' (Gunn, 2001, p. 5).

In the final response, the complaints manager explains to the complainant his/her right in relation to taking the complaint further if (s)he is still dissatisfied. When this is the case, the complainant can request an independent review panel. However, the complaint can be considered at this stage only if this is agreed by a convenor appointed by a local trust or health authority. Convenors can 'refer the request back to local resolution' or 'refuse the request' (Gunn, 2001, p. 6).

Independent review panels comprise two lay people, one of whom is the chair, and the convenor, with two clinical assessors, if needed. The latter advise on complaints concerning clinical treatment and care. The panel, which is intended to be impartial, interviews both the complainant and the people complained about, and any witnesses (Gunn, 2001).

The Health Service Commissioner or Ombudsman considers complaints only when applications for Independent Review Panels are rejected by convenors, or if complainants are dissatisfied with panel decisions. Where this is the case, the Health Service Commissioner decides if (s)he should investigate. The Commissioner investigates the extent to which the complaints procedure was followed correctly, as well as the nature of the complaint (Gunn, 2001).

The 1996 Complaints Procedure has been criticised in the *NHS Plan*, which outlines proposals for reform (Department of Health, 2001). These are considered later in this chapter.

Increased complaints

The numbers of complaints dealt with by both NHS Trusts and the Health Service Commission have risen considerably (Fletcher and Buka, 1999; Hogg, 1999; Limb, 1998). There was a fivefold increase in the number of complaints received by the Health Service Commissioner from 493 in 1974–1975 to 2,660 in 1997–1998. NHS bodies received 37,350 complaints in writing in 1990–1991 and 100,033 for the financial year, 1994–1995 (Tingle, 1998a, p. 34). Recently, there have been increases in the number of complaints against both nurses (Willis, 1998) and doctors (Rhodes-Kemp, 1998; Smith and Forster, 2000). The number of cases of litigation, particularly in relation to medical staff, has also increased (Rhodes-Kemp, 1998; Smith and Forster, 2000). Some authors have argued that both litigation and complaints would decrease if clients/patients and their carers were given clear information about possible adverse outcomes and honest acknowledgement of mistakes (Allsop and Mulcahy, 1995; Smith and Forster, 2000).

The increase in the number of complaints has also been attributed, in part, to growing awareness, among the public, service users and carers of their right to complain (Elliott Pennels, 1998; Smith and Forster, 2000; Willis, 1998). This may be partly in response to patients' charters, which may raise expectations (Hogg, 1999) and the provision of more information for service users and carers by some professional bodies (UKCC, 2000a, b). In the USA:

> *A Federal Government assessment... concluded that malpractice suits are attributable to increased 'consumer assertiveness and insistence on rights, driven by rising and often unrealistic expectations as to entitlements to security and well being'.*
>
> (Smith and Forster, 2000, p. 41,
> quoting Johnson *et al*, 1990)

The Law Commission has recommended that 'corporate killing' be instituted as an offence when the death of a patient is caused by the actions or negligence of the managers of a Health Service organisation (Wilder 1999). In contrast, the *NHS Plan* proposes a 'less adversarial approach' to complaints, with resultant decreases in 'clinical negligence claims against the NHS' (Department of Health, 2001, Section 10.21).

Types of complaint

By far the commonest type of complaint in the NHS concerns lack of communication and information (Bark *et al*, 1994; Bark *et al*, 1997; Gunn, 2001). This problem is frequently mentioned in the reports of the Health Service Commissioner (The Health Service Ombudsman for England, 2000). Many complainants refer to lack of basic information: the lowest degree of participation (see *Chapter 3*). Limited, incomplete or incorrect information, particularly a lack of communication about mistakes, increases the likelihood that patients will bring lawsuits against doctors (Smith and Forster, 2000). Allsop and Mulcahy refer to the needs of patients and their families to receive 'full and clear explanation' (Allsop and Mulcahy, 1995, p. 139). Bark *et al* (1994) found in research on complainants' experiences, that patients and their carers were often treated rudely, in an uncaring way, their perspectives were ignored and they frequently received inadequate explanations.

> *... The main criticism [in Accident and Emergency and Orthopaedics]... was that staff did not acknowledge the*

patients' or their carers' knowledge of their condition and ignored information that they were trying to provide. Patients' descriptions of pain were often not believed nor taken seriously.

... Elderly patients and their carers were often not credited with any knowledge of the condition. ... Lack of respect for the patient was the most frequent complaint.

(Bark *et al*, 1994, p. 126)

Many complaints, particularly to the Health Service Commissioner, have been from bereaved relatives, partners and friends, both in relation to lack of communication and inadequate care before the patient died (Gulland, 1997; Limb, 1998; Rodgers, 1996). (See Byrt *et al*, 2002 in volume two for an example of the use of communication to empower a dying patient and his relatives.) Lack of communication with carers about the discharge of patients (Limb, 1998; Tingle, 1998b) and poor record keeping (Rodgers, 1996; Tingle, 1998b) have also been reported, as have complaints about inadequate care and treatment (Allsop and Mulcahy, 1995; Bark *et al*, 1994; Gunn, 2001). Bark *et al* report that in their study, '... in most instances (72%) the complaint stemmed from a combination of clinical and communication problems' (Bark *et al*, 1994, p. 125). In addition, many complaints concern the way that complaints themselves arc handled (Allsop and Mulcahy, 1995; Bark *et al*, 1994; Tingle, 1998b) — a point considered later in this chapter.

Responses to complaints

Research indicates that failures in communication, including lack of information, can cause (sometimes considerable) distress and dis-empowerment to clients/patients and their carers (Bark *et al*, 1994; Henwood, 1998; Royal College of Physicians and College of Health, 1998). 'A consistent message emerging from research on carers is the central importance of accurate and appropriately timed information' (Henwood , 1998, p. 27).

The quality of communication of professionals and managers and their relationship with clients/patients and their carers can be crucial in the prevention and resolution of situations which could lead to complaints (Gunn, 2001; Royal College of Physicians, 1997;

Stanton, 1997). Aspects of communication which have been stressed include taking note of individuals' perspectives (Allsop and Mulcahy, 1995; Bark et al, 1994; McManus, 2000). Williamson (2000) refers to the importance of service users and professionals working together 'towards consensus' in delineating appropriate standards of care. The need to ensure that clients/patients and their carers have a voice and for professionals to support their rights and needs, including those of minority groups (Allsop and Mulcahy, 1995) has been stressed (Gunn, 2001; Limb, 1998). The literature includes references to the need to take complaints seriously (Allsop and Mulcahy, 1995; Gunn, 2001), respond in approachable and helpful ways (Allsop and Mulcahy, 1995; Health Service Journal, 1997) and to offer apologies and explanations (Bark et al, 1997; Pickering, 2000; Smith and Forster, 2000). The *NHS Plan* states:

> *The NHS needs to be seen to say sorry when things go wrong, rather than taking a defensive attitude and to learn from complaints so that the same problems do not recur.*
>
> (Department of Health, 2001, Section 10.21)

The need for honesty and openness about mistakes has been considered earlier in this chapter. Various authors have emphasised the need for patients to have accessible complaints procedures with clear information about how to complain (Allsop and Mulcahy, 1995; Gunn, 2001) and the provision of help with complaints (Bark et al, 1994).

Smith and Forster refer to, 'an increasing public dissatisfaction with patient-clinician relationships' (Smith and Forster, 2000, p. 41). Such dissatisfaction has been found in a number of studies which have reported that some clients/patients and their carers complain of being ignored or treated rudely or patronisingly by professionals (Bark et al, 1994; Henwood, 1998; Royal College of Physicians and College of Health, 1998).

> *... Because their needs often go beyond the physiological, and include emotional, cognitive and spiritual dimensions, patients can be offended if their health professional is distant, disinterested, arrogant, shows a lack of empathy or does not extend basic courtesies.*
>
> (Smith and Forster, 2000, p. 41)

Smith and Forster (2000) argue that complaints and associated litigation could be reduced through professional codes of ethics which emphasise honest disclosure about mistakes to service users and their carers and the development of professional partnerships with them. Adequate policies and protocols concerning complaints and related education and training for staff have also been urged (Gunn, 2001; Smith and Forster, 2000; Wilson, 1998).

Complaints about complaints procedures

The complaints procedures established in 1996 have been criticised on several grounds for failing to address adequately the concerns, or meet the needs of clients/patients and carers. The lack of independence of the process, and the employment of investigating staff by trusts and other organisations complained against, has been a cause for concern (Eaton, 1998; Hutton, 2000; Moore, 1997), as has the limited granting of requests for Independent Review Panels (Hogg, 1999). In 2000, The Association of Community Health Councils in England and Wales commented:

> *It is clear that the NHS Complaints Procedures require urgent reform. We are dismayed by their lack of rigour... The purpose of the procedures must be redefined to make justice and redress for complainants the first priority. We recommend that all complaints from patients and their families should be handled by genuinely independent review panels.... All staff who deal with complaints should be clearly independent of, and trained to ensure that they behave in an appropriately fair and impartial way.*

(Hutton, 2000, p. 91)

Since this was written, the *NHS Plan* includes a comment on criticisms of the independence of complaints procedures and refers to plans to make them 'more independent and responsive to patients' (Department of Health, 2001, Section 10.21).

Although some local complaints procedures have been said to work effectively (Health Service Journal, 1997), their complex and intimidating nature has been described. Many individuals find the process of raising complaints and concerns time-consuming, requiring considerable energy at a time when they may feel particularly vulnerable (Eaton, 1998; Health Service Journal, 1997; Legge, 1997). Department of Health time-scales for dealing with complaints may be difficult to reach. The Health Service Commissioner has established a system to deal more quickly with complaints received by his office, and since 1996, for the first time, has been able to 'investigate clinical complaints' (Limb, 1998, p. 28). The role of the Commissioner has been criticised for severe restrictions in relation to the complaints which (s)he is able to investigate (Hutton, 2000). The *NHS Plan* includes a comment about excessive time taken to resolve complaints (Department of Health, 2001, Section 10.21). In March, 2001, a national evaluation of the NHS Complaints Procedure revealed problems in this area, as well as patient, public and professional views that procedures needed to be more accessible and independent, with realistic 'performance targets' and improvements as a result of complaints (DoH and York Health Economics Consortium, 2001). *Reforming the NHS Complaints Procedure — a Listening Document* includes proposals for change in these areas (DoH, 2001b). At the time of final revisions to this book, there are plans to 'provide locally based independent complaints advocacy services' in England to investigate NHS complaints (DoH, 2002).

Complaints' influence on decision making and services

Research and investigations into complaints suggest that one of the main outcomes desired by clients/patients and their carers is that complaints should produce improvements. This is frequently emphasised in the literature (Allsop and Mulcahy, 1995; Bark *et al*, 1994; Bark *et al*, 1997; Wilson, 1997). Legge (1997) reports the considerable difficulties encountered by one man in trying to gain assurance that a NHS trust had learnt mistakes in relation to the care of his mother. In one study, 90% of respondents 'wanted to prevent a similar incident in relation to their complaints' (Bark *et al*, 1994, p. 127). Cooke (1997) reported that complaints procedures were failing to enable staff to learn from experience, with a lack of feedback to professionals who had been the subjects of complaints. The *NHS Plan*, in considering future Health Service reforms, includes the comment that patients 'need to know that problems will be sorted out and put right,' citing cancellation of operations as an example (Department of Health, 2001, Section 10.20).

The rest of this chapter describes how one NHS trust took steps to take service users' and carers' complaints seriously and use them to effect improvements.

Managing complaints in North Bristol NHS Trust

A complaints manager's perspective

Complaints can provide valuable, direct feedback from service users and carers, which providers can use to improve the standard of services offered. However, the growing number of complaints in the NHS can make many staff feel threatened, defensive and protective of their actions (Smith and Forster, 2000). This can create barriers to open and honest investigation.

The approach being taken at North Bristol NHS Trust has endeavoured to change this culture. Complaints should be seen as an opportunity to use feedback to develop and improve services. Better still is the avoidance of complaints by positively encouraging patients and their carers to voice their concerns while they are still in contact with the service, either as an inpatient, in the outpatients department or within the community.

While staff have contact with the patient and his/her carers, views of the service should be solicited regularly during that episode of care. Feedback given in this way would generally be positive and a great morale booster for staff. Because criticisms are actively sought, they are less threatening to staff who are empowered to take action as a first line response, nipping potentially serious problems in the bud.

At North Bristol NHS Trust, bespoke training has been held within each directorate to discuss best practice in dealing with complaints and agree packages of training for all directorate staff. Complaints review panels have been held to look at how closed complaints have been managed and learn lessons from mistakes. Actions identified as a result of complaints are documented and progress with implementation reviewed regularly.

It takes a lot of courage for most people to raise a formal complaint about health care. The issues brought to our attention have been the 'tip of the iceberg' and we owe it to patients to take their concerns seriously and investigate thoroughly. It is surprising how many patients feel they will be 'blacklisted' as a result of their complaint, or have been scared to complain while in contact with the service. Consequently, most patients will never actually experience improvements made as a result of their complaint. This is often recognised and acknowledged by complainants, who wish to see changes implemented for the benefit of others.

What do patients want from the complaints procedure?

For most people, making a complaint about the Health Service is a scary thing to do. Many believe that the fact that they have complained will jeopardise their future health care. Complaining while an inpatient is avoided because people are frightened of repercussions and feel very vulnerable and disempowered.

Most people want to feel that their concerns have been listened to, that they will be taken seriously and investigated. They want to receive an explanation of what happened and why, in words they can understand, and, where services are not up to the expected standard, have an apology and details of the action to be taken to improve services for the future. Increasingly, patients are enquiring, some time after making a complaint, to see whether actions promised have been put in place. I think people should be encouraged to do this more often.

Good communication is essential, and complainants must be kept informed of the progress of their complaint. Failure to do so only leads to more dissatisfaction and a more difficult complaint to resolve.

Implications of clinical governance

Clinical governance in the NHS has been a major component of the changes introduced by Labour administrations between 1997 and 2002. The Government's drive to improve clinical standards is indicated in many Department of Health documents, including the White Paper, *The new NHS — modern, dependable* (Secretary of State, 1997), *A First Class Service. Quality in the NHS* (DoH, 1998) and the *NHS Plan* (DoH, 2001). Effective complaints management is an essential element in improving standards; and can enable lessons to be learned from the feedback complaints provide, in relation to the six key areas of clinical governance. The latter include clinical audit, risk management, clinical effectiveness, quality management, staff and organisational development and evidence-based medicine (DoH, 1998).

Complaints about services provide an indication of areas of risk for trusts. They illustrate areas where the quality of the service is poor, they provide an insight into training needs both across the organisation and within specific areas, and provide feedback from users about the effectiveness of the service. The complaints manager is usually the only person with a comprehensive overview of complaints across the trust and is well placed to pick up problems. Audit departments should be involved in auditing the actions taken as a result of complaints and their success in improving patient care.

The difficulties of multi-agency complaints

The public view of the NHS is a service provided across the country to treat people when they become ill, through hospitals and people working in the community. There is little understanding of the role of the purchaser and provider, the general practitioner and the interface with social services. When individuals seek help or redress from complaints, they should not be adversely affected by barriers or gaps in services. When a complaint concerns issues which cross service boundaries, it is very difficult for the complainant to distinguish where one service ends and another begins. In the patient's best interests, services should collaborate to respond fully to concerns raised, in a single response covering all aspects of the complaint in a seamless way.

Where responses are sent by each service involved in a complaint, there will inevitably be gaps in the response or areas where the sequence of events do not quite fit. Consequently, the complainant is left with an unsatisfactory answer and the dilemma of deciding how best to pursue an appropriate solution to their concerns. A valuable opportunity for working together to improve interaction between services is lost because the deficiencies and how to remedy them are never clearly identified and owned. A complaints policy developed for North Bristol NHS Trust contains a section about the Trust's approach to multi-agency complaints.

Vexatious complaints?

Some NHS trusts and health authorities have policies in relation to 'vexatious complaints', a term covering a wide range of complaints. Great care should be taken when applying this label to a complaint and it should not be one person's decision to decide that a particular complaint is 'vexatious'. In any case, what is a 'vexatious' complaint to a health service manager may be viewed quite differently by the complainant and by independent organisations representing his/her interests.

A number of instances where a complaint may be considered 'vexatious' are listed below. Many of these items are outlined by Gunn in his delineation of 'serial complainants' (Gunn, 2001; pp. 30–32). From the perspectives of Health Service organisations, it is unlikely that the label 'vexatious complaint' will be used unless it falls into two or more of the categories listed below:

- excessive persistence in pursuing a complaint
- changing the substance of a complaint or continually raising new issues or seeking to prolong contact by continually raising further concerns or questions
- unwillingness to accept documented evidence or denial of receipt of adequate response, or failure to accept that facts can sometimes be difficult to verify
- failure to clearly identify the precise issues to be investigated, and/or where the concerns identified are not within the remit of the trust to investigate
- focusing on a trivial matter
- threatening or using actual physical violence
- during the course of addressing a registered complaint, having an excessive number of contacts with the trust, placing unreasonable demands on staff
- harassment or verbal abuse, on more than one occasion, towards staff dealing with the complaint
- recording of meetings or face-to-face/telephone conversations, without prior knowledge and consent of other parties involved
- unreasonable demands or expectations and failure to accept that these may be unreasonable.

The problem with such a list is that it represents the agendas of Health Service organisations, rather than those of complainants. The categories can be differently interpreted by the service user or carer making the complaint and the personnel investigating it. For example, what is 'excessive persistence' to a complaints manager may be perceived by the complainant to be reasonable effort to obtain redress in the face of an inadequate response from an NHS trust. An apparently trivial matter or an 'unreasonable demand' to a manager may be of overwhelming importance to a service user. While organisations representing service users and carers would not condone physical or verbal abuse, this may, in part, be a reaction to failure to take complaints seriously, or to inaccessible and intimidating complaints procedures.

Some trusts and health authorities have adopted policies for dealing with 'vexatious complaints'. At North Bristol NHS Trust, guidelines were considered, as a policy was felt to be too prescriptive. In fact, very few complaints will ever fall into this category. In recommending this label, the complaints manager must be absolutely sure that the trust can do no more to answer the concerns raised and that each concern has been given fair and objective consideration. The decision to attach this label to a complaint must be taken at a very senior level within the trust and be endorsed by the chief executive and chair or their nominated deputies.

Guidelines about such complaints have not been available widely within the trust as it was considered that only the complaints manager, chief executive and chair need this information. No one else in the trust would be able to recommend that a complaint be considered vexatious, and staff would only need to know how the action plan agreed for the complaint affected them. Once applied, clear instructions must be given to any staff who are involved in the complaint or who may be approached by the complainant about the actions they should take and to whom they can refer. A regular review of this label must be undertaken to ensure it remains valid and any new complaint made by the complainant must be considered separately.

Figure 15.1 summarises what patients want, and what they have a right to expect from the complaints procedure. This list is based on work in this area in North Bristol NHS Trust, and also reflects complainants' views reported in the literature.

Figure 15.1: What do patients want from the complaints procedure?

- ⌘ Serious consideration of their concerns
- ⌘ Thorough investigation
- ⌘ Detailed response
- ⌘ Action
- ⌘ Apology
- ⌘ Timeliness in responding to complaints
- ⌘ Good communication

Source: North Bristol NHS Trust, 1999

Conclusion

Much of the literature suggests that, despite some areas of good practice, many Health Service professionals and managers have failed to take the complaints of service users and carers seriously.

Common complaints, referred to in the literature and in reports of the Health Service Commissioner, include inadequacies in care and treatment; and lack of communication, including failure to give information, or to consider the perspectives of service users and carers. A lack of explanations and apologies for mistakes has also been reported. Many complainants express the wish that health service managers and staff should use mistakes to learn and to effect improvements.

Reported problems with present (at the time of writing) complaints procedures include lack of independence; and lengthy, inaccessible, intimidating processes which require time and persistence on the part of the complainant.

In North Bristol NHS Trust, attempts have been made to prevent and ameliorate these problems. Within this Trust, good complaints management is seen as crucial to the implementation of clinical governance. It is also considered essential to deal with complaints in a patient focused way, and for the issues raised to be used to improve services. Managing complaints well can increase quality of care, improve patient satisfaction and staff morale, reduce risk and contribute to staff and organisational developments.

The publishers and editors acknowledge, with thanks, IBC UK Conferences Limited for copyright permission to publish material in this chapter previously published in Evans (2000) Managing complaints. In: IBC UK Conferences Limited *Involving Users in Clinical Governance-working with Users to Provide a Quality Service. LH 183. Conference Handbook for One Day Conference.* The Marlborough Hotel, London.

Key points

⌘ The extent that service users and their carers feel able to complain depends partly on their relationships with service providers. This has ranged from recipients of charity from superior donors to the service user having an equal or superior relationship with the professional.

⌘ Legislation for the investigation of complaints followed widely publicised scandals concerning serious neglect and ill treatment of vulnerable clients. The Health Service Commissioner post was created in 1973. However, it was not until 1985 that health services were required to have complaints procedures.

⌘ A national complaints procedure, introduced in 1996, involves four stages, ranging from 'local resolution' to investigation by an independent review panel, and ultimately, by the Health Service Commissioner if the complaint is not resolved locally.

⌘ Recently, there has been a considerable increase in complaints to local Health Services and to the Commissioner. There has also been a rise in litigation against medical staff. These increases are said to be related to raised expectations and awareness of the right to complain.

⌘ The most frequent complaints are about 'lack of communication and information'. Many complaints concern poor care and communication of patients who have died; or relate to ways in which an initial complaint was dealt with. Issues highlighted in the literature include; lack of concern for service users' and carers' perspectives, reluctance to admit mistakes, and professionals' negative attitudes.

⌘ Complaints procedures have been criticised for lack of independence and failure to address the needs and concerns of service users and carers. At a time when they are particularly vulnerable, complainants are often faced with intimidating and complex procedures. The *NHS Plan* aims to make these 'more independent and responsive to patients' (DoH, 2001).

⌘ Complainants often express the hope that their complaints will result in improvements, but frequently experience limited or no feedback about this. It is important that they are listened to, and taken seriously, with appropriate explanations and apologies, and feedback about progress in investigations. The courage usually needed to make a complaint should be recognised.

⌘ At North Bristol NHS Trust, efforts have been made to avoid the problems identified in the literature. Complaints are prevented by inviting service users and carers to express their concerns and views. Relevant staff training is provided. Managers review all complaints, which are documented, with reviews of progress, and efforts to learn from any mistakes.

⌘ Action taken in response to complaints should be audited, and used to improve standards, in relation to clinical governance; and indicate service effectiveness and staff training needs. Where more than one service or agency is involved, there should be collaboration to address the complaint.

⌘ Caution is needed in labelling complaints as 'vexatious', bearing in mind the different perspectives of complainants, organisations representing their interests and managers. Identified characteristics of 'vexatious complaints' may represent health services' agendas, rather than those of service users and carers. In North Bristol NHS Trust, only very senior managers have decided that particular complaints were 'vexatious'. Few complaints acquire this label.

References

Allsop J, Mulcahy L (1995) Dealing with clinical complaints. *Qual in Health Care* 4: 135–43

Bark P, Vincent C, Jones A, Savory J (1994) Clinical complaints: a means of improving quality of care. *Qual Health Care* 3: 123–32

Bark P, Vincent C, Olivieri L, Jones A (1997) Impact of litigation on senior clinicians: implications for risk management. *Qual Health Care* 6: 7–13

Cooke M (1997) Discounted complaints. *Nurs Management* 4(4): 12–13

Department of Health (1994) *Being Heard. The Report of the Review Committee on NHS Complaints Procedures*. (Chaired by Professor Alan Wilson.) DoH, London

Department of Health (1995) *Acting on Complaints. The Government's Revised Policy and Proposals for a New NHS Complaints Procedure in England*. DoH, London

Department of Health (1998) *A First Class Service. Quality in the NHS*. DoH, London

Department of Health (2001a) *The NHS Plan. A Plan for Investment. A Plan for Reform*. Online at: http://www.doh.gov.uk/nhsplan/npch10.htm

Department of Health (2001b) *Reforming the NHS Complaints Procedure — a Listening Document*. DoH, London: September

Department of Health (2002) *Involving Patients and the Public in Healthcare*. http://www.doh.gov.uk/involving patients

Department of Health and York Health Economics Consortium (2001) NHS Complaints Procedure. National Evaluation. Executive Summary. DoH, London: March

Dickens C (1966) *Oliver Twist*. Penguin. T Fairclough, ed. Penguin Books, Harmondsworth. (First published in monthly instalments 1837–1838)

Duxbury J (2000) *Difficult Patients*. Butterworth Heinemann, Oxford

Eaton P (1998) Clinical view column. *Nurs Times* 94(27): 49

Elliott Pennels CJ (1998) Nursing and the law 12. Complaints procedure. *Prof Nurse* 13(9): 594–5

Fletcher L, Buka P (1999) *A Legal Framework for Caring*. Macmillan, Basingstoke

Friedson E (1975) Dilemmas in the doctor-patient relationship. In: Cox C, Mead A, eds. *A Sociology of Medical Practice*. Collier Macmillan, London: chap 17

Gulland A (1997) Nurses under fire from ombudsman. *Nurs Times* **93**(50): 17

Gunn C (2001) *A Practical Guide to Complaints Handling in the Context of Clinical Governance*. Churchill Livingstone, Edinburgh

Health Service Journal (1997) Survey reveals weakness of complaints system. *Health Service Journal* **107**(5534): 4

The Health Service Ombudsman for England (2000) *Second Report For Session 1999–2000. Part 1. Summaries of Investigations Completed, October, 1999–March, 2000*. HMSO, London

Henwood M (1998) *Ignored and Invisible? Carers' Experience of the NHS*. Carers National Association, London

Hogg C (1999) *Patients, Power and Politics. From Patients to Citizens*. Sage Publications, London

Hunt G, ed. (1995) *Whistle-blowing in the Health Service. Accountability, Law and Professional Practice*. Edward Arnold, London

Hutton W (2000) *New Life for Health. The Commission on the NHS*. Vintage, London

Jones K (1993) *Asylums and After. A Revised History of the Mental Health System from the Early Eighteenth Century to the Nineteen Nineties*. The Athlone Press, London

Klein R, Howlett A (1973) *Complaints against Doctors*. Charles Knight, London

Legge A (1997) Questions of care. *Nurs Times* **93**(41): 42–43

Limb M (1998) The fixer. *Health Service Journal* **109**(5625): 26–9

Lupton C, Peckham S, Taylor P (1998) *Managing Public Involvement in Healthcare Purchasing*. Open University Press, Buckingham

MacAlpine I, Hunter RA (1969) *George III and the Mad Business*. Allen Lane, London

McManus IC Gordon D, Winder BC (2000) Duties of a doctor: UK doctors and 'good medical practice'. *Qual Health Care* **9**: 14–22

Martin JP with Evans D (1984) *Hospitals in Trouble*. Robertson, Oxford

Moore A (1997) It's no use complaining. *Health Service Journal* **107**(5561): 14

National Health Service Executive (1996) *Complaints. Listening... Acting... Improving. Guidance on Implementation of the NHS Complaints Procedure*. Department of Health, London

Perceval JT (1991) Extract from: A Narrative of the Treatment Received by a Gentleman, During a State of Mental Derangement. (First published 1838–1840). In: Porter R, ed (1991) *The Faber Book of Madness*. Faber and Faber, London: 246–7

Pickering WC (2000) An independent medical inspectorate. A proposal to promote patient benefit by encouraging medical openness and the clinical accountability of medical staff in the UK. In: Gladstone D, ed. *Regulating Doctors*. Institute for the Study of Civil Society, London: 47–63

Rhodes-Kemp R (1998) *A Remedy for Medical Complaints. A Practitioner's Guide to Complaints Procedures*. Sweet and Maxwell, London

Rodgers ME (1998) The NHS complaints system: April fool or justice for all? *Br J Health Care Management* **4**(6): 298

Royal College of Physicians of London (1997) *Improving Communication Between Doctors and Patients. A Report of a Working Party*. Royal College of Physicians, London: March, 1997

Royal College of Physicians of London and College of Health (1998) *Stroke Rehabilitation Patient and Carer Views. A Report From the Intercollegiate Working Party for Stoke*. Royal College of Physicians, London: November, 1998

Secretary of State for Health (1997) *The New NHS — modern, dependable*. The Stationery Office, London

Smith ML, Forster HP (2000) Morally managing medical mistakes. *Camb Q Healthc Ethics* **9**: 38–53

Stanton T (1997) How to avoid complaints and how to respond to them. In: Pickersgill D, Stanton T, eds. *Making Sense of the NHS Complaints and Disciplinary Procedures*. Radcliffe Medical Press Ltd, Abingdon: chap 14

Tingle J (1998a) Patient Complaints. In: McHale J, Tingle J, Peysner J, eds. *Law and Nursing*. Butterworth Heinemann, Oxford: chap 3

Tingle JH (1998b) Complaints about nurses: the unlearnt lessons. *Br J Nurs* **7**(13): 753

United Kingdom Central Council for Nursing, Midwifery and Health Visiting (2000a) *Have You Been Mistreated by a Nurse, Midwife or Health Visitor?* UKCC, London: October

United Kingdom Central Council for Nursing, Midwifery and Health Visiting (2000b) *Protecting the Public. How the UKCC promotes high standards of nursing, midwifery and health visiting care*. UKCC, London

Wilder G (1999) Dial M for manslaughter. *Health Service Journal* **109**(5670). Special report: Law: 10–11

Williamson C (2000) Consumer and professional standards: working towards consensus. *Qual Health Care* **9**: 190–4

Willis J (1998) Should nurses start running for cover from patients' complaints? *Nurs Times* **94**(15): 53–5

Wilson J (1998) Incident reporting. *Br J Nurs* **7**(11): 670–1

Conclusion

James Dooher and Richard Byrt

This concluding chapter briefly summarises the main points discussed in this book, with particular reference to the effective implementation of strategies to increase the empowerment and participation of service users and informal carers.

With such a broad range of contributors who encapsulate a complete spectrum of opinion, full consensus was never expected. Similarities and differences in the perspectives relate to personal interpretation, born from experience, and perhaps the side of the fence one happens to be standing on.

There have been uncritical assumptions that 'empowerment' and 'participation' are necessarily good in themselves. Some contributors refer to the rhetoric in many policy documents, which contrasts with the negative experiences of many service users and carers. The editors suggest that there is a need for clear conceptualisation, where those concerned develop an understanding of the level and type of cooperation that is realistically achievable. It is only then that clearly formulated principles can be generated, which may then be applied meaningfully in practice.

Higher levels of participation and most dimensions and components of empowerment involve shifts in power and ideas of equality and/or partnership. Some contributors describe oppression and powerlessness, but others give examples of successful attempts to enable empowerment and/or participation. Some examples are based on individual experience, practice or research in relation to the achievement, or the lack of it.

Professionally-initiated empowerment which produces actual change, is directly related to the willingness to share or relinquish power. Different organisational goals, organisational systems, cultures and treatment approaches seem to generate the spectrum of empowerment outcomes. However, it seems that professional attitudes and communication have some of the greatest influence upon the professional-service user/carer relationship. This relationship will be enhanced if issues such as opportunities for the person's 'voice' to be heard, information and choice are considered. In addition, control, autonomy, accessibility and advocacy including rights and the right to complain, are crucial in the development of this relationship.

Inclusion increases skills, self-efficacy, self-confidence and a sense of personal control. These components are seen as particularly important in any model of participation. Democratic participation is concerned with involvement in decision making and shared responsibility: important areas at all levels to achieve social inclusion.

Lower degrees of participation have been criticised for failing to redistribute power. However, it is argued that individuals can feel that they have power according to one dimension, but experience disempowerment in relation to others. In addition, service users and carers vary in the extent that they want different dimensions of empowerment and participation.

Empowerment and participation are affected by dominant discourses in wider society, Government and health policies, including commercial interests. It is with this in mind that the editors consider empowerment to be of limited value if users and carers continue to face social exclusion, discrimination and stigmatisation.

James Dooher, Richard Byrt
September 2002

Useful organisations

African and Caribbean Users and Survivors Forum
332 Brixton Road
Brixton
London SW9 7AA
0207 411 2944

Alzheimer's Society (Leicestershire and Rutland Branch)
204 Kingsway
Narborough Road South
Leicester LE3 2TW

Arts Action
The Orchard Centre,
14 Lothian Street,
Bonnyrigg
Mid Lothian EH19 3AB

Arts Advocacy Project
Dundee Rep Theatre
Tay Square
Dundee DD1 1PB

Art in Hospital (Glasgow)
Blawarthill Hospital
129 Holehouse Road
Glasgow G13 3TG

Arts for Health
Manchester Metropolitan University
All Saints
Oxford Road
Manchester M15 6BY

Bridgeton Music Project
Queen Mary Street Nursery
20 Queen Mary Street
Bridgeton
Glasgow G40

Carers National Association
20–25 Glasshouse Yard
London
EC1A 41T

Centre for Arts and Humanities in Health and Medicine
Durham University
Durham DH1 3LG

Centre for Creative Communities
118 Commercial Street
London E1 6NF

Healing Arts
St Mary's Parkhurst Road
Newport
Isle of Wight PO30 5TG

Hospital Arts
St Mary's Hospital
Hathersage Road
Manchester M13 0JH

Lapidus
Association for Literary Arts in Personal Development
BM Lapidus
London WC1N 3XX

The Listening Centre (Lewes) Ltd
(Patrick de la Roque, Consultant Psychologist)
The Maltings Studio
16A Station Street
Lewes
East Sussex BN7 2DB

Live Wire Theatre Group
Harbour House
The Esplanade
Lerwick
Shetland ZE1 0LL

Living Arts Scotland
11 Queens Crescent
Glasgow G4 9AS

Mental Health Shop
40 Chandos Street
Leicester LE2 1BL
0116 247 1525

Music Research Institute
(David Walters)
Coda Music Centre
Chewton Glen Farm
Highcliffe
Dorset BH23 5QL

National Arts Therapies Research
Committee
BCAT
The Friends Institute
220 Moseley Road
Highgate
Birmingham B12 0DG

National Association for
Poetry Therapy
#280, 5505 Connecticut Avenue NW
WASHINGTON, DC 20015
USA

Poetry Therapy Research
(Dr Robin Philipp)
Centre for Health in Employment
and the Environment
Department of Occupational Health
and Safety
Bristol Royal Infirmary
Bristol BS2 8HW

Positively Women
347–349 City Road
London EC1V 1LR
0207 713 0444

Project Ability
Centre for Development Arts
18 Albion Street
Glasgow G1 1 LH

Rethink Severe Mental Illness
(Formally: National Schizophrenia
Fellowship)
30 Tabernacle Street
London EC2A 4DD
0207 330 9100

Specialist Dramatherapy Service
Dundee Repertory Theatre
Tay Square
Dundee DD1 1PB

Stimulating Creativity
Highlands and Islands Arts
Bridge House
20 Bridge Street
Inverness IV1 1QR

Survivors' Poetry Scotland
30 Cranworth Street
Glasgow G12 8AG

Survivors' Poetry (UK)
Diorama Arts Centre
34 Osnaburgh Street
London NW1 3ND

Survivors Speak Out
34 Osanburgh Street
London NW1 3ND

Tamalpa Institute (for expressive
arts therapy)
PO Box 794
Kentfield
California 94914
USA

Therapeutic Writing — Stories at Work
Institute of General Practice and
Primary Care
Sheffield University, Community
Sciences Centre
Northern General Hospital
Sheffield S5 7AU

User Voice
Ten Acres Centre
Dogpool Lane
Stirchley
Birmingham B30 2XH

Index

C